FUN DIET

It's Not *What* You Eat, It's *Why* You Eat

Andrews, Ryan

FUN DIET: It's Not What You Eat, It's Why You Eat

/ Ryan Andrews – 1st ed.

ISBN 978-09983068-1-0

Printed in the United States of America

Design by DreamSurf Studio

FIRST EDITION

To my wife Nissa,
who never stops believing in me;
and our four amazing children.

CONTENTS

A NOTE TO MY READERS

I wrote this book with one goal in mind, to change the conversation when it comes to diet, weight loss, and those of us who have been stuck with more weight than we want. The current landscape for weight loss is all about selling products and pushing a new technique on us. Everyone who has ever lost a lot of weight and kept it off can tell you that the system they used wasn't nearly as important as how they changed on the inside during that process.

I have been obese and know the shame of being heavy. I understand the embarrassing things that we go through just to live in a world that thinks we're lazy and lacking self-control. Having conversations with someone who has never struggled is just an exercise in frustration.

The *FUN DIET* is designed to bring a breakthrough, not weight loss. Your weight is a byproduct of your biochemistry, diet, exercise, and consistency. There are lots of methods, products, and tricks that can be used to lose weight, but there is an entirely different method for never having to struggle with weight ever again. The goal of this book is to break free from the shame and the struggle of dieting and to remove the stuff blocking ultimate freedom. I still go up and down with my weight like an average person does, but I'm never stuck. I am a healthy weight for my size and it's never a struggle to make good decisions and fit in the same size clothing year after year.

I may not be a doctor, nutritionist, psychologist or biologist but I am a guy who has conquered the weight demon in my own life and has helped other people do the same in theirs. Please check what you read in here with your health professional. There are some techniques that may cause a conflict with the medication you're taking or if you're getting help with mental health, some of my suggestions could trigger you if not discussed with your provider. Nothing in here is extreme and for the vast majority of you, the information and advice are exactly what you need.

I am an avid researcher and studied numerous white papers, studies, and techniques from the world's brightest cutting edge providers. I am the best-selling author of the book, FUNDAMENTAL: The transforming Power Of Having Fun, in which I utilize many Positive Psychology techniques to teach the process of enjoying life.

Breakthrough happens in a moment, but it might be decades in the making. If you're truly ready to be done with the diet yo-yo once and for all, then you're reading the right book. May God bless your journey and may you find peace, joy, and hope.

When you get your own breakthrough moment I would love to hear from you. Let me know about the things that impacted your life. If you need any encouragement or help, send me an email or connect on social media.

At the end of each chapter there are notes and helpful worksheets. If you need a place to write something down, look there first.

God bless!

FACEBOOK

www.facebook.com/fundietbook

WEBSITE

www.Ryan8.com/fundiet

PRIVATE SUPPORT GROUP

www.facebook.com/groups/fundiet

Chapter 1
THE FUN DIET

You are not **what** you eat,
you are **why** you eat

Diet is a 4-letter-word for: torture yourself physically, mentally, and emotionally. It's synonymous with "I'm admitting to all my friends, family, and coworkers that I know I'm overweight and I will 'try' one more time to prove that it's not possible for me to be thin." It has become an annual torture test by way of the New Year's resolution and is almost as touchy a subject as politics.

Mosts diets begin with high hopes that this will be the one; only to be rejected by the difficulty of living on planet earth while following the directions. Or it is so expensive that the credit cards are maxed out, the freezer is full of food that will never be eaten and there's a tub of ice cream calling out, "I'm ready when you are!"

Diets were meant to be broken! It's not possible to sustain a diet because the rest of the world isn't doing what you are doing. The purpose of most diets is to get you "thin" quickly and then get you into a normal routine of healthy eating and regular exercise. If you're not starting out a diet with the understanding that you are planning on changing your life forever then most likely it will be another failure.

Here's the good news, the FUN DIET is a completely different look at what it takes to live the life that you want all while being a healthy weight. For some of you, this journey is a struggle with 10-20 pounds, while others it's a battle with 100-200 pounds. If you're stuck, regardless of the total weight, then it can feel like an impossible uphill challenge. The aim should never be to lose weight. The aim should be to get healthy and let the weight take care of itself.

HOW CAN A DIET BE FUN?

The top question I get asked when I mention The FUN DIET is, "How can a diet be fun?" Often it's followed up by, "I'm on a diet, and it is definitely not fun!"

The Answer: If the diet you are on is exciting, and adds to your overall enjoyment of life then it will be fun!

A diet is not something you go on to get thin, it is supposed to be how you live your life. If the diet you are on isn't something you can sustain for the next 40 years, then you might as well quit now. Our weight is a reflection of how we eat compared to the level of exercise we do and all of that is hidden behind a wall of stress, shame, fear and anxiety. It's all about why we choose poorly even when we know the right things to do.

WHAT IS THE FUN DIET?

The Fun Diet is a completely different way of getting a lifetime of healthy weight. This is not just a diet. Through helping myself and others slay the weight demon once and for all I have discovered that there is so much more to it than a simple nutrition and exercise program. I share my struggles, reveal the shame I dealt with, and open my heart for you all to see the process, so you can get the same breakthrough I had.

Nothing good is ever easy, but everything worth fighting for is good. The weapon of choice is "having fun and enjoying life." The impetus is that life is too short not to live it on our terms. The goal is to dream big and enjoy the process.

The fundamental principle of this program is that people are not heavy because of what they eat but WHY they eat. Many programs work: counting calories, "carbs are the enemy," drink coffee with butter in it, score points based on the food you eat. The list goes on and on, and every diet program works. Well, they work for some better than others, but all of them show results. I have found that there is ONE HUGE thing connecting all of these diet programs, they focus more on the WHAT than the WHY.

My body chemistry is different than yours, and lifestyles dictate what our nutritional needs are. Where we live, the level of stress in our lives, and our gender all require slightly different nutritional needs. Some diets will help you lose weight, but the result could be a vitamin B deficiency which can lead to depression. If you live in the north, the winters are relatively severe and low on sunlight so some diets could cause a person to gain weight where the same person living in Florida, for example, may experience a total body transformation. There is so much more to being a healthy weight than what the scale reads or what your pant/dress size shows.

Starting with WHY helps put in context what the actual health needs are of an individual and sorts out what type of a diet they should be on. This diet works along with any other program on the market; the goal is that you will be forever free from the shame and struggle of weight and that you would find life enjoyment. That seems like a lot for a diet program, but it's what I have achieved, and I know you can have the same.

WHO IS THIS FOR?

The Fun Diet is for anyone who feels stuck with their weight or overall body health. I have seen some lose hundreds of pounds, and I've seen others get rid of that last 10 pounds of stubborn weight. Surprisingly it's the same process and the same types of things that help both. The outside is a reflection of the inside. This program is for anyone who has ever felt shame from the diet yo-yo or has dreaded seeing old friends or family because of their weight or how they look. If you have ever worn a t-shirt in the pool, so you don't get made fun of or if you've ever said the words, "I can't be thin" then this book is for you. If you are anything like me, you've been happy being heavier and never considered it to be a problem but deep down you wish that it didn't have to be that way.

Most of the testimonials I receive are different than your typical weight loss program, and I want to share some with you here so you can see what you're about to start. Here's one from a group program I developed.

"He quit the job he hated, and picked up his guitar and is teaching music. He is currently down to 192 lbs. (lost 25 pounds)"

Notice that this testimonial talks about finding passion and removing something that he was stuck behind. After the shift, then he lost 25lbs which was more than his initial weight goal.

"…is happy; she is now a runner and very HAPPY with her physical strength and the fact she sees herself much more confident and capable. (She has lost 15 pounds!) Not to mention the fact she is challenging herself to do things she never thought possible."

I love this testimonial because it has nothing to do with the weight. This woman has what she's been after, happiness with herself. How many times do we put ourselves down or think bad things about ourselves while looking in the mirror or trying on clothes? The goal of being a healthy weight and overcoming the struggle and shame of the diet yo-yo is so we can look in the mirror and be happy with what we see. At the time of this printing she hadn't reached her final weight goal yet, but her life is changed forever and reached a goal that she never planned on, "doing things she never thought possible." I know as she continues to pursue her core identity the weight will continue to melt away.

"There are more lessons to learn, more vulnerability to embrace and lots of miles to cover! I really appreciate the time you took to sow into our lives."

As you can see with these testimonials, the impact of The Fun Diet is more about enjoying life than it is about losing weight, as it should be. The more connected you are to the awesome power of your own life the more your physical body will reflect that. Here's one more that I LOVE:

"Writing down my "why's" has made a real

difference. I haven't changed anything in my diet except for the journaling. That alone has made me stop and think before automatically going to the fridge. That seems to have been my nemesis, grabbing something to eat when I am bored (not hungry). Also, I have a number on the scale that I have not been able to get below. Every time, I've gotten down to this number (but no further), I'd think that if I could just lose even a 1/2 lb. I'd be over that block. Yet, the next day I'd be right back up. (It sounds weird, but it's been my truth for a long time.) In the past 5 days, I have gotten past that number and continued to lose."

This woman was in a wheelchair and struggled for a long time. Today she has completed a Spartan race, 5k run and is working towards a ½ marathon and is continuing to lose weight. Every day you can see her light shining brighter and brighter.

I love this story because she found a group to work out with and now has a support group that will see her all the way to the finish line. Ultimately we can be, feel, and do anything that we want but connecting with our heart is the key to all of it.

HOW DOES IT WORK?

There are three major pieces to the puzzle. BE yourself, FEEL alive, and DO life. The third one is the most recognizable; I call it the

"DO" phase and it's all about technique; nutrition and fitness.

Often times if we're in need of losing some weight it's not that we're stuck but more that we just need to stop eating junk and start being physically active. The DO (technique) is what we're used to seeing with diet programs. It includes the: how to, education, and practical steps to losing weight.

The second part is the "FEEL (mindset) alive" phase which tackles the mental aspects of doing something different and challenging. What you've been doing in the past hasn't been working, so we will be doing something else moving forward, and that challenge is mentally challenging. Learning how to have the mental fortitude to overcome weight challenges will be one of the keys to lifetime success.

Our primary piece of the puzzle is a big one, BE. This is your core identity and the lens through which you see yourself. In this part, we tackle the real reasons you have struggled and been stuck for as long as you have. Without really going after the truth of WHO YOU ARE, it's tough to have lifetime results.

THE FUN DIET IN A NUTSHELL

The *FUN DIET* starts with preparing to tackle nutrition and exercise by working on the reasons why we are stuck, next we build our strength and resolve through mental exercise and emotional balance, then we find foods that are exciting and methods of exercise that are fun and add those to our lives. The decision to remove the things that are stealing joy, and taking away from reaching our goal is not part of the program; those things will naturally fall away.

JOIN THE PRIVATE FACEBOOK GROUP

Studies show that having support or joining a team helps people be more successful than if they went at it on their own. Because of this, I created a support community of Fun Dieter's who understand where you're at and have read the same stuff you have. Together is better than alone. Come join the group and start sharing your goals, struggles, successes, and wisdom.

FACEBOOK GROUP:
www.facebook.com/groups/fundiet

My Goals

_____

_____

_____

_____

_____

_____

_____

_____

_____

_____

Chapter 2
MY WEIGHT JOURNEY

The man in the mirror is now a champion of my soul instead of the bane of my existence.

C oach shouted at me half joking, "Andrews, GAIN SOME WEIGHT!" I was the number one starting defensive end on the varsity football team of my high school, and I was a great player. It was my sophomore year, and I had just finished a good practice. The weekend before I had one sack and a defensive touchdown. The problem was I weighed 150 pounds, and I was playing against guys who were 275 pounds. If a team decided to run a bunch of blockers at me followed by the guy with the ball it was tough for me to hold my position because of my light weight. I shouted back, "YES SIR!" and promptly gained 70 pounds in about three months.

That's right, seventy pounds in only three months. I ate peanut butter and banana milkshakes all day long including my regular massive food intake. I started working out every day, and as luck would have it, I grew 3 inches in that time as well. It was the perfect storm of a growth spirt and massive calorie intake combined with regular heavy weight lifting. I still have the stretch marks on my shoulders, legs, stomach and butt to prove it.

Gaining weight and bulking up lasted the remainder of my high school football career. I toned down the PBB shakes, but I still ate anything and everything that I wanted. What I didn't realize is I was creating a mental marker that made an emotional trigger which built a habit. I was stuck, and after football, I continued to gain weight and live the life that I created for myself.

One day at the gym I stepped on the scale, and I was 280lbs. It was the first time in my life that I ever considered that my weight gain was out of control. And it was the first time that I ever felt shame because of how I looked.

Shame was not a part of my training; this was all new for me. Growing up, I had lots of self-confidence, and I love myself. I learned how to strut my stuff no matter what stuff that was, and I was good at everything. I was a star athlete, 3.6GPA student and I was friends with just about everyone I met. Shame took me by surprise.

I did what anyone else would, I went on a diet. It was more like I went on a cut out everything fun in my life to grind my way down to a "healthy" weight program. I started running, and I hated running. I removed all treats and cut back on my overall food intake. Believe it or not, I was very healthy in what I chose to eat at meal times. Growing up, my parents were big into health food. I was even a strict vegetarian for a few years in middle school. Healthy food might be better for your health, but it is still full of calories like everything else so eating a lot of healthy food will still cause weight gain.

I felt great! I lost 30 pounds and was happy to be bouncing around the 245 to 255 weight range. During my time after football I had started lifting heavy weights and I had quite a bit of muscle mass. That was my excuse anyway. Yes, muscle weighs three times more than fat, but even with my muscle mass, I should have been no heavier than 225 if I was a healthy weight.

People commented about how they could "really see it in my face." I had accolades for losing weight, and getting "fit." The praise felt good, and I was back on top of the mountain again. As I slowly gained the weight back little by little, the accolades stopped, and the shame crept it's way back. I remember getting out of the shower and looking in the mirror..."What a fat ass!" I said aloud to myself for the first time. The mirror became a source of pain for me every single day. "There he is again, the fat man in a little mirror." Over and over every day of my life I would say horrible things to myself because of my weight.

Going clothes shopping was a whole new experience for me. What do you mean I need to get a size 46 pants I'm a 36 dammit! The shame of that new suit hurt badly. I was still a 46 long, but for the first time in my life, the tailor had to let the pants out, not take them in. "What have I become..."

You know how it is, not every time and not everyday but often the shame would creep in and bury the real version of me deeper and deeper under a smothering layer of fat. Holidays would come around, and it was time to break out the fat jokes from friends and family. Then prove them right by eating four plates of food at Thanksgiving and downing six helpings of dessert and washing it down with a quart of eggnog. I liked to joke about my weight and make everyone laugh. No one was ever mean to me, except for the man in the mirror. That guy broke me down every day.

It hurt when someone else reminded me that I was heavy, but it hurt worse when I felt like this was how I was going to be for the rest of my life. I went back and forth like that for a long time. I would lose 20 pounds then gain it back. Holiday season was great fun; I got to break out my fat pants and enjoy some good food. Then January first would roll around, and I would hate myself though another diet program.

It was always about the weight. It was always about being fat, and not fitting in my clothes right. The clothing industry doesn't like heavy people. A larger version of skinny pants doesn't work when you're overweight. My calves and quads were way too big. I had to get pants where the waist was huge and baggy just so my ass fit in them. Putting on a fitted shirt only accentuated my belly, and if I got something that fit it was like wearing a tent.

WHAT HAD I DONE

During my bulking up days for football I had created a mental marker by associating gaining weight with success. It was positive for me to be big enough to throw my weight around. It was a sign of doing well to eat whatever I wanted, and eating had become a reward for working out hard. All of that made an emotional trigger for me that whenever I was feeling like a failure, I should eat. Whenever I was stressed, I should eat because it will make me feel good. And on the opposite side whenever I did well I should celebrate with food. Food had become something bigger than nutrition it had become an addiction.

The natural part to eliminate is the habit of eating large quantities of food. Most diets focus on creating healthy habits, and those are good, but they are not the real problem. The habit is a result of what emotional triggers exist and the lens that is used to view life. Habits take 21-28 days to create and 2-3 times longer than that to break so if you've ever been on a diet for longer than 30 days you created a new habit. The reason that habit didn't stick is that it didn't address the real issue.

Over and over again I broke my habits. I would create a habit of eating poorly and not taking care of myself physically; then that practice would lead to a new diet or exercise program. I would break that habit then create another healthy one, then break that one and create another unhealthy one. The cycle would continue this way, over and over. That created a myth which grew with every passing year, "I was big boned, and being heavy was how I was born."

Even though I was always thin as a child and both my parents were an average healthy weight, somehow in my brain, I believed that I was big because of genetics. It is true that the men in my family history are great at putting on muscle mass and we are all big people. What isn't true is the lie that my genes made me fat. I promise, I'll get into this later, but for now we continue the story.

THE PROBLEM

Everyone needs an outlet. If you don't have an outlet for your emotions, then you are like a water balloon stuck to the spigot, at some point, you will pop, and it will be messy. One good outlet is exercise; there are few better forms of an emotional release than to exercise. Other kinds of bad outlets like alcohol bring a slight release from the emotional build up; it's more of a reserve tank than an actual outlet, so the temporary relief only adds to the pressure for a later time. A good outlet equals actual emotional release. A bad outlet equals dump emotions into a reserve tank for a later explosion. We eventually deal with all emotions either today, tomorrow or way in the future but we do deal with them.

My outlet of choice was food, specifically sugar and fats. I love cookies and pastries and doughnuts oh my. One year for my birthday I requested cookies instead of cake. When I'm depressed, I need a dozen doughnuts or a pint of ice cream. When I'm celebrating, I need a dozen doughnuts of a pint of ice cream. It doesn't matter what the occasion is, but it has been my downfall from day one. I crave the sweets.

At the same time, for my main meals, I would choose creamy or cheesy things when I'm in an emotional crisis. We call them comfort foods, and there is science as to why we crave fatty foods when we need "comfort" but whatever the reason is, I love 'em.

The result of this emotional buildup is fat on my body and a lack of motivation. I carried on my body the result of not having a proper release valve for my emotions. Every time I had problems paying the bills or relationship struggles, I would eat my way to happiness. I never really had a plan for how to deal with my feelings. Since I had created an emotional marker for success and a good outcome my default was to eat...a lot.

I had a legitimate food addiction. I didn't even know it, and if you told me that I would have laughed in your face. I mean, I was happy, and I had a good life. People liked me, and I was able to lose twenty pounds whenever I wanted to. "I could quit anytime I want." I think this form of addiction is more prevalent than we realize. The definition of Addiction is "a medical condition that is characterized by compulsive engagement in rewarding stimuli, despite adverse consequences." I would say gaining a bunch of unnecessary weight is an "adverse consequence," and a cookie is definitely rewarding stimuli!

It wasn't until just a few years ago that I had the breakthrough which led me to understand that I had a problem. Prior to that, I only "struggled" with my weight. I mean it was easy to drop some pounds when I had to, but no matter what the result was always gaining the weight back.

THE FIRST WEIGHT BREAKTHROUGH

I lumbered out of the shower one morning, wiped the fog off the mirror and began my daily ritual of berating myself into some form of sadistic motivation to lose weight. This time it worked, but had nothing to do with the horrible things I said to myself. Instead this time, I stopped in mid-sentence. "What are you doing, Ryan? You wouldn't let anyone talk to you that way, so why is it ok to talk to yourself like that?" Shaking my head like a dog drying off I said, "How does it make Jesus feel when you are talking to yourself like that? What would your wife say about it?"

I was right; there is no cause for treating myself like a bad dog. The amazing thing is that once I realized what I was doing, it was easy to see what I needed to do instead. So, I made a simple plan.

MY FIRST NON-DIET, NON-WORKOUT WEIGHT LOSS PLAN THAT BROUGHT FREEDOM FROM 30LBS FOREVER.

The plan was simple. I loved food, and there was no way I was giving up on the food I enjoyed eating. So, I made a plan to only eat one plate of food regardless of how "hungry" I thought I was. I could fill my plate to the tippy top if I wanted to, but one and done was the motto. It worked well, in the process I shrank my stomach, and within just a few weeks I didn't need more than one plate of food. Technically what it did was cut out about 2,000 calories per day. I would say that's a good start.

Step two was to cut out sugar; it was time to kill the sweet tooth. It wasn't that difficult to do. After seven days of struggle, I didn't really want it anymore. I had one rule that helped with this. If I had the munchies or was craving anything sweet I was always allowed to have a piece of fruit.

Step three is one we utilize for the Fun Diet because it served me really well and that is to go out and play. I chose sport as my form of exercise. I didn't know how to play basketball, but my wife is a phenomenal basketball player, so I took a ball down to the local court and would run around and shoot for 30 min every day for lunch. Eventually, I found a group of guys that didn't mind me making mistakes and let me play with them. Every Tuesday and Thursday I played basketball for 1hour during lunch.

The result of this was I lost 10lbs. the first week and 30lbs. by the end of 3 months. Over the next six months, I didn't lose 1 pound. I had hit a plateau, but it didn't matter. I was having fun playing basketball, and eventually, I got invited to play soccer as well, so Monday and Wednesday I played soccer and Tuesday and Thursday I played basketball. In the past when going on a diet, I would have ended my program during the plateau season and been satisfied with my results. I also would have gained it all back shortly thereafter.

The difference was that I was having fun. I didn't cut out anything from my diet that I enjoyed eating beyond sweets and quite frankly those are unnecessary. I added exercise but because I was having so much fun playing soccer and basketball it wasn't a workout program that had an ending. I just kept playing!

Once that plateau was over, I had lost around 60lbs. I was thinner than I had been during high school (post growth spurt) and felt better than I ever had before. After this first breakthrough, I only ever gained part of the weight back. I had overcome one of the great hurdles in my life; believing who I am at my core is not dictated by what I do and how I look.

MARRIAGE, KIDS, AND STRESS

As time went on and I started to have children, slowly, the weight crept back. I never got huge again, but I definitely gained enough weight back to feel bad. It was easy to blame it on "sympathy weight" that I acquired with every pregnancy, or I could have chocked it up to getting older. I slipped back into some bad habits, but the reality was that I was stressed out to the max with financial struggles and I defaulted back into my old mode of food as an emotional release.

I had developed my "DO," the technique that worked for me with diet and exercise but as I slipped out of that technique I gained the weight back. I never let it go all the way this time. I was able to maintain a level of discipline because I liked how it felt when eating healthy and smaller quantities. It was fun to try new foods, and I was more conscientious about what I was eating.

The big difference this time, I was a lot easier on myself. The guy in the mirror had learned his lesson, and he was no longer beating me up for gaining weight. Even though gaining weight was a struggle, I knew that I had a plan that would work whenever I was ready to go for it. Just having that in the back of my mind made it easier to come back from packing on a few extra pounds.

For years I went back and forth with a 10-pound fluctuation balancing around 240lbs. I would gain weight during times of stress, like the end of the month when the bills were due. Then lose it again when I started to feel myself slipping away. For the most part, I was happy with my weight, and I was alright with being a "big" guy.

Four kids later, I had some balance to my life financially, and the significant stresses were mostly temporary or typical business related. I had returned to playing soccer as my form of exercise, and life was good. Still, I was stuck. I was eating right and exercising regularly, but for some reason, I wasn't losing any weight. The answer was fairly obvious based on my current diet but more complex than just what I was "DO"ing. The BIG BREAKTHROUGH came in the form of a midnight diaper run and what transpired after.

THE GREAT CINNAMON BUN DEBAUCHERY

We had just run out of diapers, and I was tasked with running to the store to make sure we had some for when the baby woke up. It was late, and I was irritated by having to get dressed and go out when I had already snuggled up on the couch to watch a movie. Being the good husband I was, I jumped up and headed to the store.

I had created a bonus system for when I had to do something like this. Treat time! As a "reward" for going to the store late to get diapers, water, other food, or whatever the family needed I would pick out my favorite treat and enjoy them before bed. This time was no different.

I had the diapers in hand but what treat to get was taking longer than normal. Maybe I wanted ice cream... or doughnuts... or perhaps some cookies??? Then they revealed their goodness to me like finding the holy grail. Shining like a beacon on the shelf was a dozen cinnamon buns. BINGO! That's what I was looking for but was torn about getting the whole dozen. I only wanted one, well really I wanted three, but I certainly didn't want twelve. "Oh well," I thought, "I can share some with the kids tomorrow." I gathered my treasures and headed home.

On the car ride home, I ate 2 of them. I noticed all the lights were out, "I guess everyone went to bed." I sat down on the couch with another cinnamon bun and started the movie I had left hanging on the TV. SIX more buns later I began to feel a little sick from all the sugar. I thought, "I have to destroy the evidence. I should take these to the trash outside. Nissa will be disappointed in me if she sees how many I ate." On the way to the garbage, I ate the rest of them.

I tossed the tin in the trash and tail between my legs I headed back inside and plopped down on the couch. "I can't believe I ate them all! What did I just do?!" The shame of what I had just done settled onto me like a bone-chilling fog. I went back and forth with myself like Smegal and Gollum from *Lord of The Rings*. Finally, I reached the point where I thought to myself, "Ryan, you have a real problem. You need to get professional help."

In the morning I found my wife in the kitchen and sheepishly confessed what I had done the night before, "Last night I bought a dozen cinnamon buns, and ate them all; I think I have a real problem." She laughed. Not a judgmental laugh, or a mocking laugh, her laugh was simply, "I love you, and I don't have a problem with you, but if you need help I'm here for you." She said all that with a simple laugh. I told her that I thought I needed to get some help and she just supported whatever I thought I needed.

By the time we finished the dreaded conversation, I felt great inside, and the weight of my situation had lost all its power over me. I decided I would do a simple juicing reboot. My plan was to juice carrots for breakfast and make a green juice for lunch then eat a healthy dinner. Again, I cut out all refined sugar. The plan was seven days of that, then reassess what I needed to do.

I felt so great at the end of 7 days that I continued for 30 days. I augmented the plan a bit and started eating something for lunch, but I still juiced both breakfast and lunch. I also missed having pancakes with the kids on Saturday mornings, so I added that back in as well. During that time I took a business trip to Detroit and even while there I was able to continue the plan without any problems.

It's easy to be on a diet when you enjoy what you're doing. For me, I felt so full of energy like never before that my morning juice was more important than the average person's coffee ritual. I loved it, and I enjoyed what was happening inside me. Sixty days later I was still doing it. I had lost 20lbs, and I wasn't even trying to lose weight. I was in between soccer seasons, so I wasn't even exercising.

A friend of mine who is also named Ryan, was great at asking deeper questions about what was going on with me beyond the surface diet issues. As we talked, I realized that during those last

60 days, I had been doing a lot of soul-searching and spent lots of time digging into the core of who I am. I started to bring to light all the good things inside me. I wasn't focused on the weight or any of the negative thoughts that I struggled with on that fateful night of cinnamon debauchery.

I was having fun with my nutrition and exercise. I had connected with my "Who Am I" like never before. I was working hard at that time, but for some reason, the stress and emotions that had plagued me in the past were being dealt with better. I was in communication with my wife about my feelings, and I was honestly taking internal inventory on a regular basis. The man in the mirror was now a champion of my soul instead of the bane of my existence.

I had broken free. I felt it. Food was no longer my master. I was no longer a slave to food as an addiction. I had found the way out, and it was to go inside. I learned how to feel again.

What Are Your Favorite Comfort Foods?

Chapter 3
THE FUN PART

Once you've unlocked what's really keeping youstuck, the weight melts away.

THE FUN PART 33

Have you ever started a diet thinking, "I can't wait to cut out all the food that I like to eat!" Or have you ever said, "I'm looking forward to punishing myself daily," I hope not! If you've ever been excited to start a program, it's because you believe that it's going to solve your problem forever. The method in this book, BE - FEEL - DO, will provide the tools necessary to have a lifetime of a healthy weight but even with that if you're not having fun then you probably won't even finish the program. One of the biggest challenges with diets is that they're not fun at all!

Life is short. No one wants to spend their entire life eating things they don't like and taking time away from things they like doing to grind out 5 miles on a treadmill. We do these because we want the outcome, a healthy, happy, fulfilled life. We forgo happiness today for the promise of happiness tomorrow. And rightly so, we are miserable about being heavy, or at least I was. It's worth it to do whatever it takes to be free from the shame and struggle once and for all.

Giving up what we have today for something that may or may not come tomorrow isn't always the smartest thing to do, especially when there is no end in sight. How long do you have to keep up the diet routine? When do you get to stop the exercise regimen? Is this something you will have to do every year? What about the holidays? Living a life of torture so you can stay thin isn't worth it. You would be better off overweight and happy than thin and miserable. I know many people who blow up their lives to get healthy, and it's completely unnecessary.

In business when an investor buys into something he gives up what he has, money, for the promise of something in the future, more money, but there MUST be an end in sight. There has to be a time as to when the return is going to come. It's called an exit strategy. With your dieting, if you don't have an exit strategy then you will never succeed. With the *Fun Diet*, the exit strategy is to discover healthy things that you love doing and make you come alive. The plan of action is to have fun and enjoy your life. The result is that you are living a healthy happy life, your weight isn't a concern, and food doesn't have a grip on you anymore.

Whenever we give up one thing to get another in the future, there must be some form of an endgame. With kids it's to raise happy, healthy, adults; not to provide for people for the rest of their lives. Can you imagine if a football game never ended? You would turn it off and never watch again, or if your favorite TV show ran 24hrs a day eventually, you would never want to see it again. If the end goal of a diet program is to be thin, then once that's accomplished you'll start gaining weight back until you're unhappy, then you'll try to get thin again and repeat that over and over.

Think about it, if you lose *ALL* the weight that you planned on, how confident would you be that you won't gain it all back? Losing weight isn't the issue, anyone can lose weight. Our weight is a reflection of our lives. If you have a problem with your weight, then it's likely that there is an issue in your life that needs resolution. The way to tackle this is similar to the way a firefighter puts out a fire, they remove the air and fuel from the equation, then the flames go away on their own.

That's what we're going to do, remove the problem and the emotions attached to it, then learn how to deal with our nutrition and exercise properly. Once we do that, the weight will lose itself.

Wouldn't it be better never to have to be concerned with going on a diet again?

Because the goal of this program is for you to increase your enjoyment of life and to have fun, you're not giving up current happiness to get future happiness. There will be times in the program where you may not have fun with one of the instructions, but it's not forever. It's just for a week or two, or even 30 days but that's it. Getting to the healthiest version of you should be fun even when it takes work. The result should be that you have discovered things that make you come alive, and you will choose those over the things that keep you stuck.

Ultimately you will gain a little weight because life is worth living and at Thanksgiving, I'm going to feast! But it won't trigger a downward shame spiral of consuming massive quantities of junk food. Instead, it will be a one-time event, with leftover turkey sandwiches, come Monday morning the next week you will be excited to get back to your regular eating/exercising routine.

When I travel it's been difficult to get the food that I LOVE to eat, so instead I make the experience of being off my routine as part of enjoying life. When I return, I'm happy and excited to get back to the way I like to live. The reasons we get stuck have nothing to do with food!

WHY FUN IS SO IMPORTANT

Dieting alone can cause stress which triggers cortisol so, in the end, It comes down to biochemistry. Your body chemicals can block your ability to lose weight and also can prevent you from sticking with a program. Similarly, there are others that help you stay true to a program and encourage weight loss. Learning to work with your body instead of against it is part of breaking free.

Fun is a stress reliever. There are two kinds of stress, immediate stress like playing a sport or jumping out of the way of an oncoming car, and prolonged stress like a frustrating daily tasks, relationship pressure or even being on a diet. They all produce the "fight or flight" a chemical called Cortisol.

Cortisol in short bursts is not bad for you. It's triggered to help your muscles work faster and stimulate your brain to fire more rapidly. It's closely connected with adrenaline, and it functions to keep your blood sugar levels high enough to be competitive and survive a life-threatening incident. In moments of low blood sugar like when fasting, it will help stimulate other body functions to keep you alive for longer.

When exposed to prolonged stress your immune system shuts down, and your metabolism slows. Another unfortunate side effect is bone loss. Cortisol sacrifices some of your daily body needs to provide for what you require at the moment. Cortisol creates a resistance to insulin and reduces calcium absorption in the intestine. It slows down your healing time, muscle repair, and the development of collagen which is used by muscles, tendons and joints not to mention collagen is what makes skin look young and elastic.

In layman's terms when you're stressed, you gain weight, get sick, and your body starts to fall apart.

Having fun is one of the best ways to relieve stress and mitigate your cortisol exposure. It makes sense that having a diet program that focuses on enjoying the process of learning how to stay thin and doesn't require you to torture yourself to have a successful outcome is the ONLY answer when it comes to weight loss.

SOME BRAIN CHEMICALS PRODUCED WHILE HAVING FUN:

(Excerpt from FUNdamental: The Transforming Power of Having Fun available on amazon.com)

Dopamine is a motivator for taking action. Fulfilling goals, needs, and desires produce pleasure for achieving them in the form of dopamine. Low levels of dopamine or a smaller number of dopamine receptors leads to procrastination, low self-esteem and being unhappy. If you are procrastinating, experiencing self-doubt or low self-esteem and a lack of enthusiasm, then you are probably low on dopamine.

Serotonin is considered by some researchers as the "mood chemical." If you're feeling depressed or lonely, it's because this chemical is in low supply, or your body is having trouble receiving the serotonin. It comes from feeling significant or important.

This chemical release comes from positive experiences and feelings of value. Consciously being grateful for things, Vitamin D, and having fun are all ways to boost serotonin levels. Telling stories of past experiences helps release serotonin but reliving the past in a bad way hinders your body's reception of serotonin.

Oxytocin creates intimacy, trust, and helps build relationships. It's released during orgasms, childbirth, and breastfeeding. It has been proven to help men with fidelity. One study showed that men who were given a boost of oxytocin and were in a monogamous relationship interacted with single women at a more appropriate distance than men without the boost. In general, it helps create improved social interactions. Receiving a gift raises oxytocin levels and it's fun to get and give a gift!

Endorphins are released in response to pain and stress and help to alleviate anxiety and depression. Laughter and exercise are the simplest ways to get those endorphins flowing. Even the anticipation of something funny can release them.

Pleasurable foods and smells all trigger a release of endorphins. Yep, dark chocolate, and even spicy foods are two of the biggies. Smelling lavender and vanilla or smells that recall good memories help release them as well. Being full of endorphins boost the immune system, lower stress, and assist your focus.

We must choose to enjoy the process of getting to the healthy version of ourselves. Later I will give you some nutrition and exercise guidelines which help your body work for you and not against itself.

Many of the people I coach to their healthy selves discover that often they eat because of boredom. Think about this: it's 8 pm, and you're snuggled on the couch, you put on a movie. How long will it take before you're looking for something to munch? If you had a decent dinner, and even a desert is there any reason that you should want to down a bag of chips or whatever?

The top 2 reasons people overeat are stress and boredom,

and they are not opposites like many diets suggest. They are the same problem. When you're crashing off a cortisol overload from a stressful day the last thing you want to do is be productive. You want to activate your dopamine receptors and reward yourself for surviving a life threatening day at the office. Eating activates the *reward* chemical dopamine and your brain goes into food bliss. The higher up on the scale of reward that the particular food is listed the more you will crave it. If you're like me, and cookies send you to the moon then a yummy snickerdoodle or chocolate chip is just the thing the doctor ordered. Sugar though is a quick dopamine release and a short term reward, not something that sustains long term happiness, on top of that the shame of breaking a diet or feeling like you broke a rule is worse than the benefit sugar provides.

What researchers are finding out is that slightly restricting food intake helps to be happier and enjoy the food you do eat even more! That is good news for us because I'm going to replace your munchies, and midnight snacking with some great alternatives, so we're about to make you a happier person. :)

Have you ever noticed how on the days you accomplish the most are the same ones that you get up early and start being productive right away? It's because eliminating important tasks and getting to those nagging honey do's reduce your environmental stress triggers. If you start taking care of the little things, you'll be amazed by how the rest of your world will be impacted, including your health and fitness. All of this is aimed at eliminating boredom by reducing our exposure to stress. Low stress means low boredom.

THERE IS A CORRELATION BETWEEN STORED TRAPPED FAT & STORED TRAPPED EMOTIONS!

It is important that we talk a bit about how emotions connect to habits and more importantly how they connect to weight, overeating, and being stuck. Obesity psychologist Jim Keller, interviewed 14,000 people considering bariatric surgery, and he has found that the causes of obesity are complex. "Obesity is not simply a function of laziness or an indication of emotional instability." Also, genetic and biological factors do not act in isolation but are constantly interacting with an array of environmental factors. The reasons we get stuck isn't just one thing; it's usually several different factors working together.

If you're overwhelmed, it's common for your living space to feel overwhelming. Creative types often have messy desks because they also have messy minds. Typically musicians and artists feel their way to being creative and that requires making a mess, so their workspaces will reflect that. If your life is in order and everything is going along smoothly then most likely your house is clean, your cars are maintained, and your workspace is spotless. It's true that our world reflects what's going on inside of us.

For that same reason, being fit and healthy is also a reflection of what's going on internally. In times of high stress, it's common to pack on some extra weight. The holidays are a perfect example. Most people gain the most of their year's weight during November and December. I've heard the argument that it has to do with the colder weather but why then is January the number one time of year for exercise and weight loss programs? Naturally, the New Year's Resolution drives this, but it's still the middle of winter.

The main reason people gain a lot of weight over the holidays is two-fold. Number one is the sweets, treats, and feasting! Secondly, it is the highest stress time of the year. Not only at work trying to close out the year strong but also spending money on Christmas and Thanksgiving. Then there is also the family part of the equation. Many people have stress about being around family, either because everyone is coming over to the house and it has to look like a Norman Rockwell painting or because relationships are strained. Whatever the impetus for it, the holidays trigger a mass of stress.

Internal struggles reveal themselves externally through weight, among other things. It makes sense then if we've fought to eliminate the extra weight that there is something internally that is holding us back. We can be justified in being offended or even validated by other people in not letting go, but it's worth exploring ways to overcome the sticking point.

Grief - One of the top things that keep people stuck in any area of life is grief. It doesn't have to be from the death of a loved one. Grief can come in many forms, divorce, or a strained relationship with one of your children, losing your house to foreclosure, anything that is a loss can cause grief. The greater the loss, the more powerful the grief.

In the case of divorce if there were children involved you will probably see that person for the rest of your life. Every Time you do, if you haven't fully grieved and moved on it will hurt. For our purposes, you will also not be able to let go of that stubborn, trapped fat.

Losing a loved one is another sensitive area, but it is important to go all the way through the grieving process. Deal with the emotions of the loss, and get help if you need it. Your loved one would never want your life to be impacted negatively forever because of their passing. Everyone grieves differently, so, however you choose to deal with things make sure that you deal with them. Take the time to do it well. There's no need to rush this, but the process of letting go will allow you to move forward with your life.

Regardless of what form of loss you may have experienced, taking the time to grieve properly is a key to not creating a sticking point in your life. I don't want to make light of this, and I don't want to presume to know what you've been through, but I have seen over the years of helping people, that this point is worth making.

Unforgiveness - This one isn't fun to hear, but it's true. Not letting go of past wounds can keep you stuck for the rest of your life. It can come in many forms as well. Forgiving others for things they have done to you is one of the hardest things, especially if what they did to you was heinous. You don't have a choice though if you want to move forward with your life.

It may be beneficial if I define forgiveness a little. Forgiving someone doesn't mean that what was done to you is ok. It doesn't mean that someone else is allowed to do that thing to you again, and it doesn't let the other person off the hook for their actions. It's simply a decision to not hold onto it anymore. According to the Oxford Dictionary, to forgive means to - "stop feeling angry or resentful toward (someone) for an offense, flaw, or mistake." There are of course stronger versions of forgiveness even as far as a complete pardon for the offense, but those things take time. Know that the deeper you forgive, the better it will be for you. But I say, do what you can to move towards letting go. Your life is worth healing these wounds.

One of the toughest areas of unforgiveness is forgiving ourselves. It can be just as hard to forgive yourself for messing up or doing something awful to someone else. Even if the other person doesn't even know that you did it, the guilt and shame can keep you stuck of ever. I've seen this often where people don't feel that they deserve forgiveness for their actions and it will trap them in a cycle of self-destructive behaviors.

Shame - I had so much shame around being heavy that I know this is a major sticking point for some people; it was for me. Every time I would get a little treat or order a pizza I felt shame inside for what I was eating. The crazy thing about shame is that it creates a downward spiral. The more shame you feel, the more you eat, the more you eat, the more shame you feel; over, and over, and over.

When people asked me how I could have gotten so heavy, I would talk about not having an "off" switch. "Why don't you just stop eating," they would ask with sincere intention. The truth is that I didn't want to stop eating. If I bought a bag of cookies, then that bag is going down the hatch in a couple of hours. The shame of knowing that eating this dessert is the reason I'm heavy would cause me to eat more. What difference did it make, I already started I might as well finish.

The big area of breakthrough for me was in jumping off the shame-go-round. Learning how to allow the one moment to be just that one moment. If I'm stressed out, and I want something sweet to satiate my emotional hunger and buy a doughnut, then that's it. There is no shame in it. Did it help me? Not really. On a short term basis I did get a slight stress relief, but in the long run, it did more harm than good. Either way, there is no reason to be judgmental about my action.

You're not going to get things perfect every time. But as long as you're working on getting better, then having shame about getting it wrong doesn't help. If a child draws a picture of a tree and it looks more like a rock do you punish them for their effort? Of course not, you help show them how to add branches and leaves so the next time they can get it right. Obviously, we're not children, but whenever someone is in the learning process, it doesn't help their progress to beat them up about making mistakes.

It's the same thing for getting to a healthy weight and learning how to enjoy the process. If it doesn't always go perfect, then you have to give yourself the freedom to make a mistake. Shame can be the one thing holding you back from a lifetime of healthy weight.

Unknown - There are so many unknown emotional triggers and sticking points that I can't outline them all here. Just know that there is a correlation between trapped fat and trapped emotions. If you don't resonate with any of these three common areas, take some time to think about where you might need a full emotional release. If you need to get help, do it!

Some other common emotional triggers: Unloved, Unheard, Unseen, Under Appreciated, Overworked, Taken Advantage of, Unworthy, Trapped, Pressure, Anxiety, Guilt, Low Self-Esteem to name a few.

4 PRACTICAL THINGS TO DO RIGHT NOW TO KICK START YOUR BODY

1. **Join or Create a Group** focused on the same things as you. If your goal is to get off the weight-go-round and feel good again, then it's time to get around 3-12 other people doing the same thing. You need a minimum group of 3 to make this work because it's not an accountability group, those don't work. And 12 is about the maximum number before you start to feel like you're not part of the group and just a participant.

   The key is to champion each other's victories, pull each other out of shame pits, and don't ever say it's ok to miss the group. Create a fun punishment for missing. It's important that you succeed together as a team.

   Being part of a group satisfies one of the base human needs for social interaction and is a great way to fast track your success in any area. There is something about a group working towards a common goal that helps everyone improve. The whole is greater than the sum of the parts. Also, we don't want to let each other down, so you're less likely to skip when you're not in the mood.

2. **Call it a night.** Getting enough sleep releases oxytocin and helps you "feel" good in the morning. It's easier to be happy and on task when you feel good. Get a full 8 hours of sleep tonight. One obvious function is that if you go to bed early, then you won't be awake to eat that fourth meal.

    On a scientific level getting less than 6.5 hours of sleep and more than 8.5 hours of sleep was linked to higher body fat. On top of that, they have found that keeping a consistent sleep pattern is a significant factor in lowering body fat. Sleeping also stimulates blood flow and repair of cells, so if you have a rough day, your body will thank you for the rest.

    If you're like me and have had trouble sleeping in the past, often something as simple as a glass of water can get you set in the right direction. Dehydration leads to troubled dreams, difficulty in "shutting off the brain" when trying to fall asleep and interrupted sleep patterns. Avoid alcohol because it's dehydrating, and have a full glass of water right before bed.

3. **Laughter is the best medicine!** Well, that has yet to be proven but what they do know is that laughing releases endorphins which relieves stress and depression. Endorphins also have been linked to weight loss through stimulating good feelings and decreased appetite. Laughter lowers blood pressure, and studies have shown it to burn calories as well. Wouldn't it be great if you could laugh yourself thin? Watch something funny or hang out with friends that like to laugh.

4. **Get outside!** Go for a walk in the park or if you're close enough head to the beach. Doing things outside helps center emotions

and relieves stress. It doesn't need to be physical. Sit outside with a cup of tea, or read a book. Work in the garden a bit, or head to an arboretum. Whatever your level of activity is, find a way to get outside. For me, I like to go for a long swim or big hike.

There is lots of science and studies about being outside, and it's health benefits. A simple internet search should get you ample articles on the topic. They have shown that when children even see a green space that it helps relieve ADHD. A study in the Netherlands showed that people living within a half mile of parks or green open areas have a much lower incidence of health problems.

The exercise aspect of being outside and how the sun provides much needed Vitamin-D is a part of the equation but I feel like there is a bigger less studied reason why getting outdoors is beneficial. Being indoors is safe, and can be lonely even when surrounded by people we know. But, people need new experiences and an element of danger. It doesn't have to be life threatening, but when you're outside, it's full of unknowns. Even interactions with people that you don't know will sometimes be surprising. When you get outside, it gives you a larger life perspective, and even if you don't actively do anything just being around the greatness of nature helps our bodies to function as they should.

HAVE FUN

Your life is your own. If you don't want to be thin, then you don't have to be. Your weight is a reflection of your life. If you don't feel right, then figure out why not and start taking steps to get there. There is no reason to torture yourself to be thin simply because the rest of the world thinks you should be. Having said that I don't believe that anyone heavy feels good about it.

I used to say that I liked being heavier. The rationale for me was that when playing sports I was able to throw my weight around and it helped me. Although that may have been true, I was finding the good in the bad. I feel much better today than I ever have before.

It feels good to fit in your clothes and to be able to do whatever you want. When I was heavier, it wasn't easy to bend over and pick up stuff off the ground, or tie my shoes. I didn't like the looks I got when eating junk food. I could tell people were thinking, "He doesn't need to eat that." My pain was more about the fact that I didn't like the way I looked not that some schmuck was judging me.

Being honest is what got me to the place of understanding what I wanted out of life. It's important for me to be able to run around with my kids. I love that my wife and I can go hiking or on a long walk without feeling like I'm going to die. Life is too short to be held back by being overweight.

Enjoy the process of getting your weight in order, it doesn't matter what diet you choose. Use the one in this book, or pick from one of the thousands of others but the process needs to be enjoyable. There will be times when it's tough. Anything worth doing will be challenging, but the outcome is bigger than whatever pain you're getting from the challenge.

EXPECTATIONS

I have found that there are a few things we can expect from every weight loss journey. It's obviously not the same for everyone, but this list is a basic rule of thumb to help smooth over those times when your body doesn't seem to be responding the way it should. While choosing to have fun instead of dieting, there will be times when you might be tempted to push it a bit harder. You are welcome to do that, but know the point is to enjoy all of your life, not just the next 30 days.

PHASES

1. **Initial Weight Loss** - HUGE, or feels huge anyway.

2. **The Slow Down** - This is when you're body is battling your emotions, habits, and biochemistry.

3. **Plateau** - You will plateau. It's inevitable that when going through your own weight journey that you will experience an extended time when nothing seems to be working. This is the time where you need to be enjoying the process, or you may never finish the program.

4. **Big Weight Loss** - Usually after the plateau time, all the work you put in pays off in a large dump of weight.

5. **New Life** - This last phase is when you're new life sinks in as normal and your reality. How long this takes varies by person, but if you've gone through the BE - FEEL - DO process then you should be settling into your new life and feeling good.

6. **Bumps In The Road** - Don't be discouraged by bumps in the road. It's normal to gain weight during times of stress or emotional tension. If you stick with choosing to have fun as a priority of your life these times shouldn't last too long.

7. **Breakthrough** - This can come at anytime during this process, but it's an important part of the phases. At some point, you will never be the same again.

What Are Some Of Your Emotional Triggers?

Chapter 4
BREAKING BAD

You can't break a bad habit; you must replace it with a good one.

Habit is all about patterns. In lab rats, habit is what helps them remember the pattern of a maze to get food. In humans it's not much different. Good habits help move us forward, and bad habits pull us down. What makes one person smoke is the same thing that makes another run 5 miles a day. The same part of our brain that compels us to overeat is the same part of the brain that helps us deny cravings for sweets and make good food choices.

It all happens in the basal ganglia. It's the part of your brain that deals with the formation of habits. What they haven't discovered yet, and likely never will is the part of the brain that deletes habits from your basal ganglia.

Basically it works like this: input pattern; repeat, repeat, repeat, pattern accepted. Since there is no delete button the only way to change the pattern is to overwrite it with the same technique. The trigger for your basal ganglia is either an emotion, feeling, craving, sensation, or any other function of your subconscious.

We all have patterns, and it's those patterns that govern the parts of our lives that we don't need to put much thought into. Waking up in the morning triggers my desire to have breakfast. For those who don't eat breakfast it's common to say something like, "breakfast makes my stomach hurt." Both triggers are patterns that our body has interpreted, repeated and put into practice. The best way to eliminate bad habits is to simply replace them with good habits. Sometimes the good habit will be to do nothing.

It's much easier to replace eating a doughnut with eating a stick of celery than it is to simply eat nothing. The issue with replacing something delicious like a doughnut with something not as delicious like celery is that there is a disconnect of pleasure. You received pleasure and comfort from the doughnut, and you are replacing those feelings with irritation and obedience by eating the celery. That struggle is why most diets can't work long term.

Starting something like a new diet or exercise program triggers higher brain activity to go on maximum drive, allowing you to stay focused and follow the instructions. As you start to get familiar with what to do the function moves to a pattern and is taken over by your lower brain in the form of an autopilot. It's exactly the same for good behavior as it is for bad behavior.

SUCCESS

When losing weight, you start to feel great. Chances are, you have developed strong healthy habits and the feeling of losing weight is AWESOME! Once you have done enough to feel good about how you look in the mirror the reward triggers start to fire and without knowing it those good habits that got you this far are slowly being replaced with stronger reward chemicals; and just like that, the bad habits have returned and the weight comes back.

So what do you do once you've lost "enough" weight to be happy? If we did it the right way and replaced the bad habits with good ones and have developed a strong enough 'why' for staying fit then the weight should all stay off. Once we experience success there is a marker for what is possible and a roadmap that worked previously and the power of habit kicks in and we can quickly and easily find our way back to health. Just like rolling a ball on flat ground, it's easy to move forward without resistance.

Most of the time when a diet "fails" it's because there was not a strong enough reason to continue. Unfortunately a large percentage of diets fail in the "plateau" phase. The person notices that the weight isn't coming off any more and start to slip here and there. Next thing they know all the weight is back and there is another reason for shame. It's time to break that cycle.

There is no shame in your process. Whether you lose 100 pounds in one month or 10 pounds in 10 years isn't important. What is important is that from this day forward all shame around your weight losses and gains go away. All those fit people you see on TV don't look that way 24-7 all year, every year. At the holidays it's common to put on your winter coat and add a few pounds. Where the breakthrough came for me is that in January I'm not making a resolution to lose the weight. I'm just back on my normal life food and exercise routine and in the process it takes about the same amount of time to lose as it did to gain. All without changing anything.

PATTERN INTERRUPT

The key to all this habit stuff is called pattern interrupt. You need to catch yourself doing bad habits then do something to break that sequence. Since it takes 21-28 days to create a new habit there are a few weeks where you won't be 100% successful. Create some tools now to help get your mind out of the basal ganglia and make a conscious healthy choice.

Later in this book I'm going to walk you through your first 28 days with a process that I've developed to form good habits.

But you can practice pattern interrupt right now by simply doing something unexpected. For example, the next time you are craving some junk food pull up YouTube™ and look for funny cat videos instead. You will interrupt your habit brought on by a craving and bring your focus back up to your conscious thinking mind at the same time.

If you want to read more about this, find a copy of my first book, **Fun**damental: *The Transforming Power of Having Fun*, and look for the section on "Syncopation" in chapter 2.

WHY THE FUN DIET IS A PERMANENT SOLUTION?

We are replacing bad habits with good habits, and specifically we are creating patterns of enjoying life as the tool for staying healthy. The goal isn't denial of life, it's discovering the life that has been hidden under a layer of fat.

CRAVINGS

Cravings are a result of an emotional need. Unless you're pregnant, then your body knows what vitamins and minerals it needs and those cravings are for nutrition. For the rest of us, a craving is simply an emotional need for dopamine and other comfort that specific foods bring. Here are some simple tips for getting past unwanted cravings.

1. **Don't eat around it.** Studies have shown that because a craving is your body's attempt to generate feel good brain chemicals that if you can outlast

it then it will go away. I've found that ignoring a problem is never the solution, so waiting it out is a good way to do it, but finding out what you really need is better. Stress is the number one cause, but many other emotions will trigger comfort eating. Find out what's going on. It could be you're just bored and you've created a mental trigger to eat when you're bored.

2. **Find Something Fun.** The number one way to get your body what it's really craving is to have some fun. If you can do something physical at the same time, then even better but finding something that stimulates those feel good chemicals is the primary goal.

    -   **Music** has been shown to increase happiness. Go after the happy songs and fun music that reminds you of having fun. Better would be to put on some dance music and start dancing.

    -   **Laughter** is the best way to get out of your subconscious reactive thinking and into your conscious active thinking. Watch some funny videos online or put on a funny standup routine. Whatever you choose to do, get laughing.

3. **Distractions work on toddlers and still work on adults as well.** If you can simply wait out a craving it will go away. Studies show that cravings don't continue to build and if you can ignore it for at least 10 minutes, then it will start to go away. Some suggestions are to call a friend and talk, or go for a quick walk. There is one important factor with

distraction. If you're feeling lonely then going for a solo walk won't help and will actually make it worse. The key is to find out what emotion is causing the trigger and do the opposite. If you're feeling lonely, connect with a friend. If you're feeling angry, go to the gym. If you're feeling stressed, find something fun.

There are many reasons that cravings come on from not getting enough sleep to creating habits by simply doing the same thing repeatedly. They key is pattern interrupt. If you stay up every night until 12am and at 11:30 you're hungry and eat junk food then breaking the pattern and creating a good habit instead is just what the doctor ordered.

In the above scenario, when you feel the craving go to bed. You don't need to stay awake if you're just laying on the couch watching TV. Chances are good that you're trying to avoid going to bed so the next day doesn't come so quickly. Find out why, then work towards resolving it.

If you must be awake, then instead of eating, do some exercise. You probably need energy so why not use the stored energy you have on your body. Some simple pushups, sit-ups, burpees, jumping jacks, or air squats are great simple to do anywhere exercises that will stimulate a release of dopamine and provide some energy in the form of burning stored calories called fat.

The point of this, is that there is something greater at work inside than just a machine to burn calories and use food as fuel. Humans are complex and the things that drive us are also complex. Discovering why you're having the craving to begin with will ultimately be your process for creating healthy habits. Developing good habits to replace the bad ones will ultimately cause your cravings to change as well. Instead of going nuts for some Rocky

Road ice cream, you will be craving some connection time with people, physical activity, or even just sleep.

YOUR BRAIN

The brain is complex to say the least. There are a couple of functions of it that can help you or hurt your weight loss journey. The majority of being "stuck" has to do with a disconnect between your conscious (active) mind and your subconscious (reactive) mind. When you try to introduce something new it goes through a process.

Your active, thinking, rationalizing, understanding mind receives information and it processes it through your general wisdom, knowledge & understanding. If it decides to act on it, then it will tell your subconscious to get on board so that in the future you will be able to make that good decision without having to think about it too much.

Here's a simple example: Your friend Joe introduces a healthy snack to you, and it looks strange. Green and brown with some odd smell. Your subconscious immediately reacts based on past experiences and sends the signal for you to reject it, so "yuck" comes out your mouth.

Joe explains the benefits and says, "It really tastes a lot better than it looks." So you give it a try. Your conscious mind just told your subconscious mind that it's wrong and we're going to give this thing a taste.

What happens next is where the rubber meets the road. You are introducing something new, and was told that it's good for you but you're allowing your tastebuds to be the final judge about it. Your tastebuds will react based on past experiences or a "Core Belief" that it has about certain flavors. If it tastes too much like dirt or lawn clippings then it may be rejected and Joe's power cluster will never again pass your lips. This is called Cognitive Dissonance.

Cognitive Dissonance is what happens when a new truth doesn't align with a core belief and therefore is rejected. In the above story, Joe's advice about the benefits of the health cluster were rejected because of how your subconscious was previously programmed. This applies to every facet of our lives. From how we handle relationships to how we deal with work situations to diet and exercise programs.

In my weight story I talked about liking being a "big guy." I liked the benefits of being big and strong and able to throw my weight around. Regardless of what the other information told me about how I felt getting out of bed in the morning to how I looked in clothing to how I saw myself in the mirror, the overriding core belief that I held was that I liked being a big guy. Because of that, no matter how many diet programs I went on, it was always going to conflict with that belief and therefore fail.

There is great news, your subconscious doesn't get to make decisions. It's simply reactive. You get to tell it what to do, think, and ultimately how to react. Just because an initial reaction is based on a core belief doesn't mean that you have to then act on that belief.

In order to reprogram your subconscious there are steps that need to take place. First and foremost you have to ignore what it's telling you to do and do something else. Secondly, they have found that it takes between 21-28 days to create a new habit and in doing so reprogram your subconscious. Just ignoring the craving or core belief for 28 days isn't going to get it done, you need to be proactive about creating that new core belief.

In the next chapter we're going to get into some of those functions and at the end of the book there three 28 day programs designed specifically to help reprogram your brain to overcome the weight issue once and for all.

You may need to finish the book before writing in this section, but it's valuable to write down your old core beliefs, and then write down what you want to replace them with.

OLD BELIEF

_____

_____

_____

_____

NEW BELIEF

_____

_____

_____

_____

Chapter 5
BE - FEEL - DO

BE yourself, FEEL better than ever, and love what you DO!

I t's time to slay the weight demon once and for all. Break free from the power that food holds over you, and live this part of your life on your own terms. The method I used for myself, and have used to help others break free is BE - FEEL - DO.

BE - Your core identity around weight, food, and emotional triggers. We help bring light to the negative belief systems that are keeping you stuck and help move you into a place of success. BE yourself, the real you, the part that is full of life. Once your identity is found, then the rest comes to you a lot easier.

FEEL - Your emotional connection to the things that keep you stuck and your mental fortitude. Our goal is to release you to feel alive, fully connected to your heart. It's easy to stuff emotions like a box of cookies; I help you create outlets for the emotions that make sticking with any program difficult, if not impossible.

DO - Nutrition and exercise are the core of every healthy diet. Our goal and purpose are to create a life of FUN that brings you into the health that you're after. So it should be a little tough for moments here and there, but it should also be exciting and driving you towards enjoying being healthy all without restricting the foods that you eat or forcing a killer workout program. We create a lifetime habit that you WANT to do, not that you HAVE to do.

Passion + Habit = Success - Whether it's sports, business, family, or health every successful person has a core belief about themselves that is unshakable, they are mentally tough and are willing to be connected to their emotions. They will stop at nothing to accomplish their dream. When it comes to being successful at living a healthy weight we use the same formula: Be Yourself, Feel Alive & Do Your Dream.

Begin with your core, the beliefs that make you 'who' you are. To get unstuck you will have to examine your good and bad self-thoughts. Some of the things you believe about yourself are good, and we need to accentuate them. Others that are either bad, incorrect, or downright destructive need to be eliminated. I have created a simple system to get down to the bottom of these belief systems I call our BS. This might be the most challenging part of your journey. The food and exercise part is relatively straightforward and doesn't take much training.

Getting to the core of why you're stuck without being able to talk to you will force you to take inventory of your feelings and emotions. It will force you to think about past hurts and possibly dig up some parts of your life that you've hidden. Unfortunately, those parts are the ones that are keeping you stuck.

You can will yourself thin if you want to by starving yourself and working your butt off. However, it'll be difficult, and the likelihood of staying thin are slim (pun intended ;). It's much better to have one good cry in the area of pain that you've hidden from and move on with your life. It's not that difficult once you get into it, but one person's identity issue will be different than another.

I've had many individuals who didn't have any significant core wounds to overcome but were stuck in believing that it's not possible for them to be thin. That was it; the primary belief was that their genes meant that they will always be heavy. I'm going to get deeper into genetics in a little bit, but the point is holding the belief that, it's not possible to be free from food, is a lie. Possibly it's because your whole family is heavy, or you were an overweight child, or you have tried so long to lose weight that it must be that you got stuck with the impossible to overcome gene. Whatever the reason, it's important to know that you can do this. You will do this, and you will have fun doing it!

I want to tackle a sensitive topic, but please read this with a smile because there is a light at the end of the tunnel. I've worked with people who were assaulted as a child, or young adult and from that moment on they're stuck in many areas of their life. This one can be challenging to get past because many issues need to be worked through. I do recommend with something heavy like this that you seek professional input but know that the key to your victory is on the other side of it. For some, just talking about it and connecting with the reality that this one issue could be the key to breakthrough is enough. Whatever you need to do, do it! Your life is worth it, and there is no reason that you should stay stuck because of someone else's horrible actions.Many wounds end up building false belief systems but creating new, stronger, identity is the key to breakthrough.

GENETICS

LIE: I have the fat gene, and it's more difficult or even impossible for me to lose weight and keep it off.

TRUTH: Everyone's body has been created to deal with food properly and when the right technique for nutrition and exercise is applied anyone can be a healthy weight.

There are three main body types and several body shapes, and it is true that some body types deal with weight differently. The belief that it's genetically impossible to lose weight and be thin I can debunk with one sentence. If you stop eating right now, you'll eventually die of starvation, and you will be thin when you get there. Everyone can be thin.

I by no means want to diminish the reality that you may have lived with for awhile, and I don't promote extreme dieting. Our beliefs are developed over time by circumstances, observation, and experiences so whatever you believe isn't automatically wrong. There are probably some half-truths behind these. Here's some science to help demonstrate how different body types carry mass. These are not an excuse to store fat, just an example of how certain body types gain muscle mass.

BODY TYPES

Let's get clear, your body type does not mean you are big boned, or that you are genetically predisposed to gain fat. It has to do with how your body holds onto muscle mass. Someone who is thin and doesn't show as much muscle can be just as strong as someone who looks like they are hulked up on steroids.

There are three main body types, Ectomorph, Mesomorph, and Endomorph. Each one carries weight slightly different and does affect what kinds of exercises will be better for you. These can be one reason why you believe what you do about genetics.

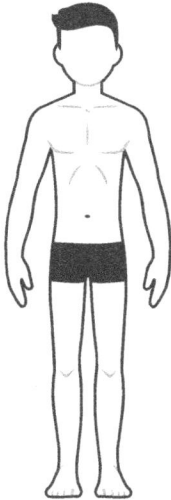

ECTOMORPH

The Ectomorph is typically naturally skinny. They are someone that can eat whatever they want and not gain weight. Their big problem is that they "can't" gain weight, which is also not true. They are thin, skinny and it's difficult to put on muscle mass. The ectomorph usually will hit a certain age where they bulk up and find it difficult to be as thin as they're used to because they have spent years eating whatever they want and not having to do much exercise to stay thin. Once the shift happens though and you start to gain weight it's simple to lose the weight again.

Focus on high calorie burning exercises like lifting weights or stair climbers and spin classes. You don't have to worry about gaining muscle mass like the other two body types, so you're free to build your strength at will. Endurance type exercise like running is always great, but you'll get quicker results out of weights or bodyweight exercises. Remember that muscle weighs about three times more than fat so as you build some muscle mass your weight exchange will slow slightly but don't worry, keep it up.

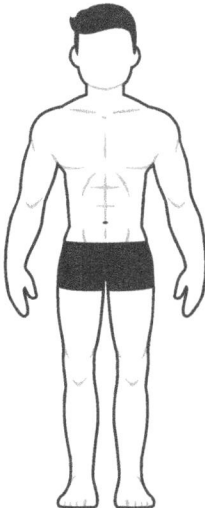

MESOMORPH

Most Americans are Mesomorphs. This body type tends to build muscle quickly and will gain fat at a relatively even distribution on their body. Since most of us, including me, fit into this category the majority of programs out there will work for losing weight and getting fit. It's just as easy for a mesomorph to gain fat and muscle as it is to eliminate it. Two weeks after not working out you will loose your fit shape and the momentum gained from it. The best course of action for exercise is to have a consistent cardio program that is fun. I like to play soccer instead of running. I still get 4-6 miles of running in when during a game, but I love playing, so it's easy to choose to do it every week regardless of the weather. Find what you love to do and do it, but make sure you focus on cardio if you're trying to stay thin. If you just want to be a healthy weight and have muscle mass, then feel free to lift weights but know that you will bulk up quickly. Most female mesomorph wonder why they can't get rid of their big legs, or overall bulk and the reason is that they are doing exercises which focus on building muscle vs. cardio. Both types of exercise are great for fat loss, and the mesomorph can transfer fat to muscle easily.

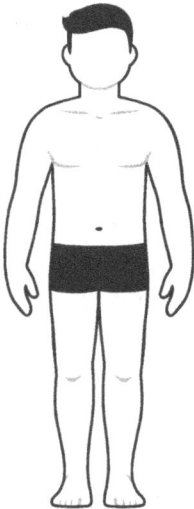

ENDOMORPH

Endomorphs would be considered stocky. Typically they are shorter and put on weight very quickly. Both muscle and fat come quickly. They tend to be strong naturally and can look heavy even when completely ripped. Robin Williams is an example of an endomorph. I use him because he didn't seem to struggle with weight issues but if you see him in movies, he would be considered stocky. Because of the ability to bulk up quickly focusing on endurance training is the best course of action for looking thin as an endomorph. The best practice though is to embrace your body type and use the ability to gain muscle as an asset. Limiting empty calorie intake will help the endomorph stay fit feeling. Using fun exercises that combine cardio and strength like kayaking and functional weight lifting will benefit the endomorph. Body weight exercises are ideal for this type. If trying to trim down in bulk focus on low weight endurance exercises.

Regardless of your body type everyone can be a good healthy weight for their body. An endomorph doesn't typically look anything like an ectomorph simply because their skeletal structure and ability to keep muscle mass prevent getting that super skinny look. There is no such thing as "big boned" so eliminate that thought.. Science only shows that there is a genetic predisposition to gain mass, not fat. Know that just because you may be more predisposed to gain muscle, it doesn't mean that you have to be an unhealthy weight.

BODY SHAPES

These are usually associated with women, but we all have a body shape that affects how we hold weight and the types of exercises that impact us.

Rectangle is balanced from shoulders to hips. The rectangle won't ever get that hourglass figure it's just not how you were made. This is the prototypical "athletic" body type and does well with complete body exercises.

Triangle is broad shouldered and typically a small butt. The triangle can have a tiny waist but because they also have smaller hips it's not as predominant. It will be easiest for this body shape to gain bulk in the shoulders, arms, lats, and back. If you want to thin out these areas, focus on leg exercises and do low weight high repetition for upper body exercises.

Pear is the opposite of triangle in that they have larger hips and narrower shoulders. It's easy for this body type to have a "booty" and thicker legs. Focusing on endurance exercise for the lower body helps with people trying to eliminate bulky legs and butt. Working heavier weight on the upper body will not typically add bulk and is a good way for this body shape to burn calories.

Hourglass has broad shoulders and back, and wide hips. Typically they have thinner waists. For keeping a balanced body with this type endurance training is best all over. If doing weights unless wanting to bulk up focus on lower weight and higher repetition.

Genetics do impact how our bodies gain weight and hold onto mass, but what it doesn't dictate is how much unhealthy weight we gain. Both gaining and losing fat works the same for every body type and body shape

BE YOURSELF

For many years I didn't feel like I was allowed to be myself, and I'm not alone. Apparently there is something called Imposter Syndrome that over 70% of humanity deals with and it's the idea that "If people actually found out who I am they wouldn't like me." It's typically associated with business where a manager or executive doesn't feel that they deserve the recognition that they received and that creates added pressure to be "something that they're not." When finding your core identity if you don't have a baseline understanding for this then you will end up falling into the "who am I" trap. I believe that Identity is one of the least trained and understood areas of life.

Who you are is something that can never change. I am a father. I will always be a father, and nothing can ever take that away. I am loved by God. Nothing I can do will ever change that. I am a man (XY). Your core personality is something you were born with but the how you've learned to behave is not. Who you are is indisputable.

Personality is another part of your identity. Having four kids, I can tell you that they are all different from each other, yet they had their personality from the time they were babies. My oldest was always a thinker. When he was an infant, he would stare at people, and you could tell he was processing what was going on. My daughter was always a goer. She walked at six months old and loved to play. She still loves to play. My next son is always smiling and is hilarious. He was a smiley infant, and always made people laugh. My youngest son is a gentle warrior. He loves to wrestle, and from the time he was first born loved to take on challenges. At the same time, he is incredibly loving and values people. You were born with your personality. You can turn those amazing traits into negative assets over a lifetime of choice and experience but the core character that makes up "who you are" is a permanent part of your identity.

I used to do this with Jr. High kids where I would get them to tell me one trait about themselves that they don't like and I would dig the gold out of it. It's a fun practice. For example the idea that I'm a starter, not a finisher was a rough one for me for many years. Once I embraced the TRUTH that I am a pioneer, then I was able to complete tasks. Now I AM a finisher, but I'm still a pioneer. I create, complete and then move forward. Another one that was negative was that I was stubborn. My grandma used to remind of that all the time. That trait is the same one that allows me to be a pioneer. I have a never give up attitude, and once I embraced it, I was able to become a do-er.

BONUS: If you're struggling with a personality trait that you exhibit and you're having trouble seeing the good side of it, send me a message on one of the social media platforms, and I'll interpret it for you. Every negative trait has a good root to it and is core to who you are. The negative qualities that you're exhibiting because of it are learned behavior. - **Facebook.com/fundietbook**

THE MAN OR WOMAN IN THE MIRROR

Both figuratively and literally when we are staring in the mirror, we can bring life or death to ourselves. The wisdom of King Solomon says, "Death and life are in the power of the tongue, and those who love it will eat its fruit." It's time to stop it! You don't have to switch right away from saying bad things about yourself to spouting positivity, but anyone can catch themselves saying something negative and stop it.

It's simple to recognize if you were to say that same thing to someone else out loud would it be hurtful regardless of the "truth" behind it? So many people say, "I'm just being real and telling it like it is." That is complete nonsense you can see things from a positive side and a negative side, so if you chose to say something hurtful, then you're mean. It's time to start being our own champions.

I used to call myself "fat-ass" and "lardo" among other worse things. I would look in the mirror and tear myself down. There is truth in those thoughts, I was very heavy and was carrying an extra 50+ pounds of fat, so it makes sense. However, I am not fat. You are not fat. Fat is not a permanent condition. Your identity is not a "Fat Person." You have the power and have the ability to be thin. When you finish this book, you'll also have the tools but if you get ONE POINT out of this whole thing pay attention here.

There is no such thing as a fat person, there are only people who are fat!

You are a person, not a fat person. You may be currently "overweight" or "heavy" or pick your politically correct version of saying that you're not the healthy weight that you want to be, but no one is a FAT PERSON.

You get to create the version of you that you want. Some have put themselves in a tight spot because of years of doing things wrong, but there is nothing that can keep you from how you want to be. I have worked with people in wheelchairs that were able to take control of their weight and health and love the new life they created for themselves. Even to the point of getting out of the wheelchair. There is no such thing as a point of no return. If you are willing to start speaking life over yourself instead of death, then you WILL see a permanent change.

I have many testimonials of people who were doing the first week of The Fun Diet, where we ask that you DON'T change any of your eating or exercising patterns, and they lost more weight than they have doing other diets. It's amazing what you can accomplish with just canceling the self-hate festival.

USEFUL SCIENCE FOR POSITIVE SELF-TALK

Barbara Fredrickson has researched self-talk in the area of positive psychology. She studied five groups of people by showing them five different emotionally triggering video clips:

Group 1 - Joy

Group 2 - Contentment

Group 3 - Neutral

Group 4 - Fear

Group 5 - Anger

After watching the clips, each person was handed a piece of paper with 20 lines on it and was asked to imagine that they were in a similar situation to the clip they watched and to come up with options for how they would have handled it. The Fear and Anger groups wrote the least and the Joy and Contentment groups wrote the most.

Negative thoughts and feelings have a positive function. If you're alone in the woods and a bear steps onto your path the fear you feel allows you to focus on one task, survive the bear! The negative thoughts limit a person's options to what they can see in front of them. Positive thoughts, on the other hand, allow the person to see more options and creative solutions. But wait, there's more!

Positive emotions increase the ability to build life skills and resources to use later in life. A kid who plays outdoors running and climbing trees and playing with friends develops skills. Running and moving builds athleticism, playing with the other children helps with social skills and making up games and using their imagination builds creativity. When a kid isn't having fun and starts to pout, they lose the desire and willpower to be friendly and play.

According to Fredrickson, this is the "broaden and build" theory. Positive thoughts and feelings widen the sense of possibilities and open our minds to see the value in what assets we have and how to use those to our advantage. Thinking negative on the other hand helps to narrow our options and limit our creativity so we can survive the bear attack.

When staring in the mirror and talking negatively about ourselves, we are limiting the possibilities to create healthy patterns and even the desire to eat healthy. When you're in the fight or flight mode, you tend to crave comfort foods and would prefer to hide under a blanket on the couch.

THE POWER OF THE MIND

All this positive self-talk brings up the second part of the *Fun Diet* - FEEL alive. How we feel impacts our ability to be mentally tough and push through when we don't feel like doing the right things to do. Feeling alive is like having the power to accomplish anything. Nothing seems impossible, and even those things that we don't like doing can get done quickly.

One of the things I started doing for fun is triathlons, which came a few years after my breakthroughs; and I was tricked into it... kind of anyway. My brother phoned me up and asked if I wanted to do an Ironman race with him. My immediate response was, YES! Shortly after hanging up I thought, what have I just agreed to do? I write about this experience in depth in my other book, *FUNDAMENTAL: The Transforming Power of Having Fun*, but there was a point during the race that I thought for sure I would have to quit.

I had completed the 1.2-mile swim, 56 miles on a road bike through the mountains of Lake Tahoe and was 1 mile into the half marathon portion when disaster struck. My right knee gave out, and I hit the ground. I was still 12 miles from the finish, and I had my family waiting for me. I got up and soldiered on with a new strategy. Walk up the hills, run down the hills, and limp jog on the flats. That worked for the next three or four hours then, BAM, the other knee gives out! I hit the ground again, but this time defeat started to sweep over me.

There was no way I was going to finish. I didn't feel like pushing any further, and I had thoughts of failure and defeat. Then, like a rescue helicopter in the middle of the ocean dropping a lifeline down to a shipwreck survivor one thought saved me. Ezekiel wouldn't quit. All of my kids are full of courage and inner strength; they are just like their mom that way, but in that moment I remembered how Ezekiel won the "Rudy Award" in football. He was the smallest kid on the field almost every time he played. He was outweighed and undersized yet for some reason the kid just wouldn't quit. They put him on the defensive line going against the very biggest kids on the field and yet he still would win and get tackles and sacks and create fumbles. He was a beast on the field, yet he was the smallest. In that moment of defeat, I pictured my children and wife waiting for me at the finish line. I couldn't quit. I can't give them permission to give up when things get hard. Ezekiel wouldn't quit.

I dusted myself off, and through excruciating pain, I continued with my plan. Walk the uphills, run the downhills, and limp jog the flats. For the next 8 miles, I drew from the mental strength I had acquired during my training. When I didn't feel like getting up at 5 am and running 8 miles I did it anyway. When the fires came through, and the air was full of smoke, I still had to train, and I did it anyway. I created space for myself to be successful during that one moment when quitting was a very real and acceptable option.

There will be moments during your weight loss journey that you may struggle to push through the "plateau" or you get set back by a week of binging from a stressful life situation. But during those times, you need to have trained your mind to get you back on track quickly. There is nothing fun about failing. Every time you quit a diet or gain all the weight back you create mental triggers confirming false beliefs about who you are.

In those moments that it's difficult to FEEL alive you will need to rely on your mental fortitude to bring you back. The power is all in being connected to your heart. I classify the heart or soul as your *Mind, Will,* and *Emotions.*

The Mind is our knowledge and understanding. It is the central computer for how we internally process all things externally. It is responsible for creating the lens by which we see the world.

Our Will is the conscious and unconscious part of our psyche. It is in charge of our deliberate actions. While the mind holds the lens for our psyche, the will holds the mechanisms for how we act and react.

Emotions are the "feelings" part of us. When we feel sadness, joy, remorse, peace, calm, stress, etc., those all belong to our emotional being.

During the FEEL portion of the *Fun Diet*, we work on creating the appropriate lens for how to filter the emotions that we feel. In turn, this helps to create the correct actions and reactions with our nutrition and exercise. Using the foundation of proper identity we create real connections to our heart, including finding strong "*why's*" like I had with my Ironman experience. Then in moments of difficulty or even failure, it's easy to come back to who we are and quickly start feeling alive again.

Find your superpower and discover what makes you come alive. Once you do that, your life will begin to fall into order. The weight will melt away, and you will start to discover activities and food that you love. During the Mindset Training, I give you some tools for finding passions and dealing with tough emotions.

ACCENTUATE THE POSITIVES

HOW does one stop a bad behavior when the mind is fighting against them? There is a simple, and complicated, answer to that question. The simple answer is just to stop it. Ultimately that is what will happen, but the path to get there can be challenging.

The complicated answer is that it takes building up to it. The battlefield is the heart. It's the negative self-talk that creates space for failing. When you say something like, "I'm bad at this," or "I can't stop doing…" or "I'll never…" your body responds in kind. You don't need to lie to yourself and say that everything is going to be ok if you know it isn't, but you can find the good and think about those things.

If for example one of your habits is eating late at night and you can't seem to kick it the negative self-talk can continue to keep you stuck. A good thing to think about is how well you did during the day eating healthy. If you went for a walk or spend time exercising, you can think about how amazing that was. This seems simple, but the more you ignore the negative thoughts and actions and replace those with positive ones the easier it will be to break the habit that has been keeping you stuck.

"Above all else, guard your heart,
for everything you do flows from it."
-King Solomon

It's important that we take care of ourselves. It's so easy to say and do things that would be unacceptable to say and do to someone else but is entirely acceptable to say to ourselves. Why? If it's a horrible thing to say out loud to another person, then we should avoid it for our own self-talk. Guard your heart and make it a rule that you will never treat yourself worse than you treat others.

The golden rule is do to others what you would have them do to you. The golden rule for The Fun Diet is do to yourself what you would do to others. Right now commit to focusing on the positives, and treating yourself like royalty. Negative self-talk is not acceptable. You deserve all the love you can give yourself.

THE DO

The reason for losing weight and getting healthy is to enjoy life to the fullest. We just went through some of the keys for how to get the breakthrough, but the reason for all of that is to have fun and truly come alive. So the last thing we want to do is kill all that momentum with a restrictive diet and brutal exercise program.

You gotta have fun! Discover new foods, and find fun things to do for exercise. Some people find that they love going to the gym, but that's not me. I love being outside, so playing sports like soccer are a big part of my personal physical exercise. I also discovered that I enjoy triathlons, especially the swimming and cycling part, so I train my swimming and cycling, but I only do running when training for the next race.

A lot of people find that they love to run so don't rule it out until you give it a good try. I don't mean once on the treadmill, but get yourself a good pair of running shoes and find a partner and start jogging until you can have a good sample size.

Hiking, walking, yoga, spin classes, and Zumba are all exercises that suit different people's personalities. When it comes to finding fun things to do, try it all! We take the same tact for nutrition. The food you choose to eat should be something you enjoy. Going on a zero carb diet would drive me insane. I'm not saying those diets don't work. I think most diets work, but there are a few that my body wouldn't like.

I love to eat bread, flatbread, tortillas, muffins, rolls, and buns. So instead of restricting my diet I create a plan. If I go out to eat dinner, I have a roll. It's easy enough to have one and done; I don't have to gorge myself. Another bad habit that I still hang on to is eating late at night. When I'm slimming down for a triathlon, then I cut this out, but I like to have a little snack before bedtime. Don't get me wrong; it is a bad habit, but because I'm not trapped by food anymore, I might go weeks without eating a fourth meal. The point is that you don't have to eliminate all the bad things you eat all at once. As you get healthier and start to find exciting new foods to eat and enjoy the bad stuff doesn't hold the same appeal as it did before.

Start with the simple things that are obvious. NO SODA! For most people, if they eliminate soda from their life they will lose 5% of their body weight within the first month. Having said that from time to time, I'll enjoy a home-brewed ginger ale. It's not about being restrictive, but we need to be smart. Chips and snack foods and desserts are obviously not going to help you lose weight. We'll get into this more in the chapter about nutrition, but for The Fun Diet, we're trying to create a lifestyle that we enjoy.

SOME FUN TIPS TO ENJOY THE PROCESS

Don't Look at the Scale - "A watched pot never

boils." From time to time, it's fine to check your progress, but looking at the scale on a consistent basis will do more harm than good. I recommend once a month as maximum, but it's not a rule just a suggestion.

Relax - If the goal is to have a lifetime of healthy weight, then there isn't any reason to hurry to get there. If some of the changes you make result in substantial weight loss then it's a bonus. There is no pressure to lose weight, only to get breakthrough. Focus on solving the problem, and the weight will take care of itself.

Have Fun - The more fun you have, the easier the process will be. Fun things to do can double as exercise. Finding fun fruits and vegetables to try double as healthy meals and snacks. Get together in training groups and find friends that are working to achieve the same thing as you.

Challenge Yourself - We all love challenges, and it's an easy way to do something difficult for short periods of time. Juicing, No Sugar, and Exercise Challenges are all examples of things that will be very beneficial but can be tough to complete on a long term basis. There are a few different challenges in this book but if you want some extras, check out www.ryan8.com/fundiet.

Life is worth living well, so even though there will be challenges along the way, there is no reason to make food a big deal. The less we make food an enemy or a hero, the better life will be for us. Food is fuel, and it's delicious. Some foods support your body functions better than others, but that doesn't take away from the power of enjoying what you're eating.

Exercise is the same thing if it's so difficult to do then eventually you will stop and starting again will be tough. Enjoy whatever season you're in and find fun things to do in that season. You will have to be intentional about finding those things to do, but you'll start to get in rhythm, and it will be easier to find exercises that you enjoy.

It's all about enjoying your life and having fun!

FUN THINGS TO DO
OR
FUN THINGS YOU WANT TO TRY

Chapter 6

NUTRITION

Extreme dieting is horrible for your body, we focus on the good things and how to enjoy what we're eating; don't force it.

In the sea of conflicting nutritional information, there are some things we can all agree on; Junk food is bad for you, causes cancer, promotes cellulite production and offers almost no nutritional value whatsoever. Having said that, there are times where a donut must be eaten just for my own sanity! You can cut out all junk food consumption, and you'll probably lose 5% of your body fat in 1-2 weeks.

The Fun Diet philosophy with foods that are not good for you is simple. Keep them to a super low minimum, and you should be okay. I've been there before when going to a party or office get together and there is nothing that you're allowed to eat. Consuming massive quantities of sugar and saturated fat isn't good for losing weight. Perhaps you don't have a ton of junk food, but you do that one bad thing every day, then I say keep it if you're ok with the damage it's doing to your body. There is no reason to eliminate things that bring you joy or emotional release unless the outcome of that thing is destructive to your life.

A good example is morning coffee. I know many people who MUST have their morning cup-o-java. Even though the caffeine in it isn't great for you and there are healthier ways to get that fix and still get your early morning smile on. Until you are in a place where it's worth doing something different, then keep it with some modification. Step 1 starts taking it without sugar, and I don't mean switch to some fake sweetener. I mean get used to enjoying it unsweetened. The point is that I'm not into sacrificing emotional stability to shed 2-3 pounds of fat. If, that one cookie you eat with your lunch every day, is part of getting your fix, then don't eliminate it right now. You can do it later when you have the proper tools.

What you'll find is that the healthier you get, the easier it will be to stop doing things that aren't serving you. All habits can be resolved. The best way to stop doing something is to simply stop doing it. Statistically, cold turkey is the only effective way to break a habit. The way to eliminate the dependence, however, is to get your identity in order and use your superpower of feeling alive to help kick the cravings and bondage to it. So we want to focus on building your internal mechanisms for living the life you've always wanted.

THE SCIENCE OF FAT

Fat is one of the three primary macronutrients, along with carbohydrate and protein. Meaning your body needs fat, carbs, and protein to survive. One of the foolish things about restrictive diets is they starve the body of nutrition that it needs to survive. The thinking is that if you don't provide fat that the body will use the stored fat but that's not how it works. Your body needs a balance of nutrition to perform different functions. It requires glycogen, which is the stored version of carbs, for quick energy and muscle function and it needs fat for prolonged activity and brain and organ function.

If you eat a fat rich diet, then your body will use the fat in the food instead of the fat on your body. The reason why diets that focus on using fat instead of carbs for energy work for a time is that you are eating fewer carbs and starving your body of glucose and glycogen. That is not healthy! Your body needs to have a balanced meal. If you consume only protein and fat, then it will use up all your stored energy in the form of glycogen, and you will be on the verge of passing out. It's true that your body will eat itself to get the nutrition it needs, but that is also not what you want. When you stop one of those diets, the body is incredibly grateful and replaces all the used up fat and glycogen as quickly as possible. In layman's terms, you gain all the weight back quickly.

Fat stores all kinds of things in it. All the fat-soluble vitamins like A, D, E and K, are saved there but so are medications. When you're sick, the body can trap the excess bad stuff in the bloodstream into fat cells to deal with them on a more balanced level.

4 FOOD RULES THAT WILL SERVE YOU

RULE ONE: If it grows in nature and it's edible then it's probably good for you. Fruits and vegetables are cancer fighting, fat fighting, and great for your gut health. Whatever you do, learn to LOVE your grown foods. You cannot eat too much fruit and vegetables the upsides far outweigh anything negative that may exist.

If you've ever been on the diets where you've been told to limit fruit and vegetable intake, then the Fun Diet is the exact opposite. I can't tell you how many people say not to eat fruit because it's full of sugar, or not to eat an avocado because of the fat. Let's stop all the pretending right now. NO ONE IS OVERWEIGHT BECAUSE THEY EAT TOO MUCH FRUIT! Sure, if you're training for a bodybuilding contest then carbs are the enemy, but for the rest of us, the benefits of fruit and vegetables are amazing.

RULE TWO: Eat the real stuff, no diet or low-fat foods - If what you're eating has a "diet" version of it then it's probably not good to be eating in the first place. Fake sweeteners are terrible for you. Not only do many of them cause cancer but they trick you into a false sense of being healthy. Also if your goal is to eliminate the sweet tooth, then it's important that you start choosing unsweetened versions.

With no low-fat foods, it's more about avoiding the versions of foods that specifically market "low fat." Milk, cheese, yogurt, and butter are all the better for you with all their fat in them. The fat will satiate you better, and you'll eat less of it. Also, the low-fat and nonfat versions are higher in the natural sugars that help baby cows gain weight. Here's a little perspective for you. Whole milk is 3% milkfat, so there isn't that much difference anyway.

We're trying to avoid being on a diet; we are building lifetime health. The fat is where most the vitamins and minerals are stored. It's also where the hormones and antibiotics are stored as well so whenever possible opt for hormone-free milk products. Fat-free or low-fat foods will often use some other product to replace the fat that they removed so going with the most natural forms of food will serve you.

Bonus: No Margarine or fake butter. Those are usually air spun canola oil or worse and those cheap oils are horrible for your body. Just stick with the real stuff, and your body will thank you.

RULE THREE: Eliminate Soda and all sweetened drinks from your daily routine. I love a good home-brewed style ginger ale but for most people trying to lose weight the enemy is a sweet tooth. Drinking sweetened drinks, not naturally sweet drinks, cause your brain to crave more sweet foods. Sodas, diet sodas, and sweet tea are some of the worst culprits. Your body will thank you for cutting back to 2-3 times per month maximum. I recommend treating sodas like cigarettes, they are killing you and are your enemy when trying to get healthy.

The average person will drop 5-10% of their total body weight by just eliminating soda or sweet tea. Let's not forget the 1000 calorie trips to Starbucks as well. That venti caramel frappuccino has a massive amount of calories and is loaded with sugar. If you need an afternoon pick me up, eat a piece of fruit. If you're stuck on coffee or tea, then get something unsweetened.

RULE FOUR: One and Done - can save you from overeating. I started this during my first breakthrough. I used to eat 2-3 plates of food for dinner, or if I ordered fast food, I would get 2-3 burgers or whatever. The rule is that you can have one of whatever you're getting. Even it's not ideal for you, one will only hurt a little. When piling my plate with food, I'm free to pack whatever I want on it, but then that's it. If I'm forced to buy fast food, which is more often than I would like with young kids in traveling soccer, then I get one big burger, burrito or whatever instead of several smaller ones. The psychological advantage is in not being restrictive and having a ton of "do not's". The physical advantage is in saving thousands of calories that your body doesn't need and won't process well.

If you're trying to kick the carbs for whatever reason, one roll or piece of garlic bread is good, but 2 or 3 or 6 is not. Personally, I don't have a problem with carbohydrates because without them we will die but being excessive is just self-sabotage. It's good to eat the way that you want all while being smart. If you only want to eat chocolate cake, then I can't help you. There has to be a desire to be healthy and to learn how to enjoy healthier options. Taste buds are all new every ten days so changing what you "like" to eat is not terribly difficult. There are psychological connections to flavor profiles, but regarding not liking broccoli or something healthy, it's only a matter of time before that will change.

NUTRITION MYTHS

MYTH: Eating a fat rich diet makes your body use stored fat instead of carbs for energy.

TRUTH: Eating fat rich foods instead of carbohydrates only makes your body starve for carbohydrates. Your body can only create triglycerides from your stored fat as a replacement for the glycogen that it stores from carbohydrates. These are not a replacement for glycogen or the glucose that it gets immediately from carbohydrates. Whenever you starve your body from something it will go into conserve mode to keep you from starving to death and does the exact opposite of what you're trying to accomplish. Eating a balanced diet of carbs, fats, and protein is important to be healthy and have a lifetime of healthy weight.

MYTH: All sugars are the same, avoid all sugar including fruit sugar and honey.

TRUTH: Not all sugars are created equal. There are refined sugars that are free from any nutritional value and there are natural sugars that are usually connected to vitamins and minerals. Refined sugars are already extracted from the plant for you and natural sugars are ones that your body needs to extract on it's own. White sugar will convert into fat in your body as soon as you're done using it. Whereas, a piece of fruit your body will convert the fructose into usable, storable energy in the form of glycogen and the like. Honey is also not a refined sugar and although maple syrup is boiled down it doesn't have the same cancer causing properties of refined sugar.

If you must, select refined sugar above fake sweeteners and other "sugar replacements." The better option is to eliminate as much sweetened foods and drinks from your diet as possible. If something is naturally sweet like an apple then it's in the "good" category but if you're drinking soda or sweet tea on a regular basis then you're just sabotaging your body. Replace refined sugar with honey whenever you can in recipes and sometimes, just cutting the sugar content in half is a good option.

MYTH: Skipping meals saves calories and is good for weight loss.

TRUTH: Skipping breakfast is the single worst thing to do if you're trying to lose weight. If you don't change anything about your diet but you add a small breakfast within the first hour of waking up you will lose weight in the first 2 weeks of doing this. The reason for breakfast is specifically because it get's your metabolism going for the day. If you skip breakfast then your body is still in starvation mode from the night before. Skipping lunch or dinner can have a similar effect. Your body needs to have a consistent intake of energy or it starts to go into fasting mode and it starts conserving energy and storing fat. If you can't get a meal, then have a snack.

MYTH: If you eat organic food then you will lose weight and get healthy.

TRUTH: Food is food. The benefit of organic is just avoiding pesticides and bad farming practices but an organic cookie is just as bad for your waistline as a non-organic one. The upsides to shopping organic is that those foods tend to use less preservatives and avoid bad sweeteners like high fructose corn syrup. But, if you're eating organic junk food it's still full of empty calories just like the regular stuff. In conclusion, go organic for your health but you still need to eat right for your body.

MYTH: Avoiding carbohydrates will help me lose weight

TRUTH: Your body needs carbohydrates to function. If you don't provide carbs then it will use up your glycogen storage and the process of doing that releases water. The result is a quick loss of weight which is mostly water weight. The downside is two fold, your glycogen storage is depleted and your body will need to replace those as quickly as possible and the other is that you lose water from your body which is a key lubricant for all joints. Basically a carb restricted diet will cause you to drop weight in an unhealthy way and when you go off that diet it will gain it all back quickly.

MYTH: Avoid nuts because they are fattening.

TRUTH: Nuts, seeds, and fatty fruits like avocado and coconut are extremely healthy for you and actually provide a great source of unsaturated fat that your body needs. In 2003, the FDA approved a health claim for seven kinds of nuts stating that "scientific evidence suggests but does not prove that eating 1.5 ounces (45 grams) per day of most nuts as part of a diet low in saturated fat and cholesterol may reduce the risk of heart disease." Coconut oil has been shown to prevent early onset of Alzheimer's and avocados are a superfood that you could literally live on. On top of all that, nuts, seeds, avocados, and coconuts have Omega-3 fatty acids which are great for your brain function and other major health benefits.

TIPS & TRICKS

Knowing what foods to eat or avoid can take time to grasp fully, but with The Fun Diet, we practice this: Relax. Do what you can, when you can and work on changing the things that aren't serving you.

Late Night Eating: Best practice is to stop eating or snacking after your last meal of the day. Also, your last meal of the day should be a minimum of 2hrs before bedtime. I understand though if you have dinner at 5 pm and you're still awake at midnight that you've gone 7 hours without eating. Our bodies like to eat a meal every 4 hours so by 9 or 10 o'clock it's very tempting to eat something, you're hungry!

> **Solution 1** - Hot liquid satiates hunger so drinking some herbal tea, or some other hot liquid can help you avoid eating. But remember, this is The Fun Diet and I would rather you enjoy your night then force a rule. Plan on making this, a bonus not a rule.

> **Solution 2** - Eat your dinner a little later. If you know, you're going to be up late then eat a full meal closer to bedtime.

You're better off having a light snack at 4 pm then eating at 8 pm if you know you're going to be awake until 12 am. The best option is to go to bed by 10 pm and finish eating by six or seven, but life isn't always ideal.

Solution 3 - Plan your dinner better. If you know, you won't be able to avoid the 4th meal then have a lighter dinner and make the 4th meal light as well. Eating late isn't all about calories, it's about "why are you up that late?" If something you're doing requires you to be awake and attentive that late then your body needs the nutrition. If you are laying on your couch watching TV trying to avoid going to bed so the next day comes slower then you may have other things to work through. The ultimate goal is to love your life!

Discover new foods - It's easy to get stuck in a routine, especially with what to eat. We eat a complete balanced all organic mostly from scratch diet, but there are days that we'll eat vegetarian or vegan. When I trained for my Ironman race, I trained all vegan. Try it all; there are great meals and different regional cuisines that are good for you and can bring some excitement to your meal planning.

Indian Food is not difficult to make, but the spices are different than the typical American spice rack. Most people find that they love Indian food even if it looks a bit intimidating at first. Go to an Indian restaurant and see what you like, then try making it at home.

Italian Food is way more than just pasta. Some of the seafood dishes are amazing and very healthy for you and your waist. Look outside the box when thinking about eating Italian food.

Mediterranean Food is some of my favorite because of the range of flavors and styles that it encompasses. Think olives and feta cheese with a bunch of fresh herbs, vegetables and fish. There is much more to it than that, but going Greek or Moroccan is very fun.

Asian Cuisine is more than just noodles and broth. Thai food is my favorite of the bunch, but Japanese style sushi, Korean BBQ, and Vietnamese spring rolls are all amazingly unique. You could get lost in all the various styles of food from the Asian region so if you're looking for something new and exciting try something other than fried rice and chow mein.

South American Food is vast and diverse. In the US we're used to getting good Mexican food if you're close to the border, but there are amazing unique cuisines that span the entire southern continent. Chilean kabobs with chimichurri sauce, Baja-style street tacos, and Gaucho style BBQ just to name a few variations.

Get out of your comfort zone and make discovering new foods a fun task. You could spend time just getting into the various American foods and still find more than burgers and BBQ. It's easy to get in a rut with our meal selections so spice it up and try something different every week!

Shop The Perimeter - This is your best bet for getting food that is going to help you and not hinders your quest for a lifetime of healthy weight. In a grocery store, they host all the fresh foods around the perimeter. The more you can cook your own meals the better it will be for you. Buying pre-packaged food of any kind will have stuff in it that you really don't want. You also don't get to control your portions, and it's often easy to overeat. Focus on buying fresh foods and skip the pre-packaged stuff.

Snack From Scratch - If there is no quick meal in your house then you will always have to make it yourself or eat a fruit/vegetable as a snack. If I'm motivated enough to make cookies from scratch, then I figure it's worth the reward of eating them. Air-popped popcorn is a good healthy snack. Not that microwave stuff or bagged popcorn, but plain kernels in an air popper is a great snack. Carrots and hummus, sliced apples and peanut butter, nuts, and dried fruit are all great quick snacks that aren't pre-made with a bunch of junk in them that you don't want.

Give Yourself a Break - A big part of being healthy is not to be too strict. Taking your time, and learning what you like to eat and the way you like to live is a major step in taking back your life. Don't waste time feeling bad about making a nutritional mistake. As we talked about earlier, if you emotionally need a piece of chocolate then you're better served eating the chocolate than stuffing the emotion. Take the time when you make a poor decision to find out WHY but don't beat yourself up over it. Relax, this is all about enjoying your life, not forcing it.

New Foods To Try

Chapter 7
EXERCISE

Life is too short to miss out on having fun because we are not fit enough to participate.

Exercise and a healthy lifestyle are the cornerstone of every diet on the planet. Supplements & weight loss gimmicks still list exercise as an essential component to the successful use of their product or program. If you asked your average person if they exercise enough most of them would answer, "no." Why?

The excuses come out of the woodwork when asked why we don't exercise. There is a lot of fear, shame, and negative thoughts surrounding exercise. Gyms are intimidating, going for a walk outside can be dangerous these days, and with the massive increase in back pain, autoimmune diseases, and debilitating weight issues the prospect of getting your sweat on can be daunting. Why we don't do the things that are clearly good for us and will prolong our life has to be due to the perceived pain of doing it is more that the pain of staying the same.

THE WAY TO OVERCOME ALL OF THIS IS WITH FUN!

Life is too short to miss out on having fun because we are not fit enough to participate. How many times have you watched friends or family have fun playing around and know that if you try to join it's just going to be embarrassing and you'll probably get hurt anyway?

Avoiding exercise because it isn't fun or we don't feel good enough is the excuse, but the real reason is likely to be much deeper. That is the catch 22 of exercise; you won't be able to participate in the things that require some degree of fitness. The solution is finding things that are fun to do and plan them as your form of exercise.

- I don't like to run, but I love to play soccer! So I get 5 miles of running in every time I play.

- I love to swim! If I hadn't started training for a triathlon, I wouldn't have found that out.

- Hiking is so fantastic for my soul that going on a 10-mile hike is a blast and also a ton of exercise.

- I love to play with my kids, so running around outside playing tag, throwing the football, or aggressive 2 square in the driveway are all forms of exercise that get's me going.

Most people don't even take the time to try new things out, so they never know what they're missing. I have one client that discovered Crossfit and became a diehard fan. I've done my weightlifting when younger, so it doesn't appeal to me as much anymore. One woman that found an early morning group to workout with at the gym, and she wouldn't miss it for the world. I just tried a spin class the other day and had so much fun that I will add that to my normal exercise options.

If you search youtube for "Arthur's Inspirational Transformation!" you'll see a man with crutches who is quite a bit overweight filming his journey trying yoga. The end is an amazing transformation where he doesn't need the crutches anymore to help him walk. He has lost a bunch of weight, and he's obviously emotionally more balanced.

That doesn't come from going to a yoga class. It's a desire to finally change and do something that is going to both challenge and inspire. The best way to stick with an exercise program is to have fun doing it.

It's easy to get in a rut with exercise. Most people don't even know what to do. They start walking or trying to jog and quickly lose interest. My mom walks like a machine, but she always goes somewhere with a view, a park, lake or the ocean. You never know what you'll find that you enjoy. One of my clients discovered chopping wood, and he thrives off it. He started a very part time wood business so that he could cut down trees and chop wood.

If you don't enjoy your exercise routine, then you won't stick with it on those days when it's inconvenient or difficult. I love playing soccer so much with this specific crew on Friday mornings that I show up regardless if it's 40ºF and raining or 110ºF and blistering hot. The most unused piece of equipment is the treadmill. How many people buy one for their homes and then let it collect dust in the corner. If we're honest, it's because it can be crazy boring. On the other hand, my friend's wife set hers up with a tv in front of it, and she watches her favorite cooking shows while running like crazy on her treadmill.

FUN IS THE KEY TO CREATING A LIFESTYLE OF BEING FIT AND ENJOYING EXERCISE.

You may find rock climbing is exciting, or like my mom you may love walking. That woman walks a ton of miles every week. Getting together on a team or in a group is one way to be excited about exercising. Even if it's not something you would do on your own when you're in a group, it can be a lot of fun. The social aspect of exercise is the reason why cardio kickboxing and Zumba classes were so popular. Everything can be intimidating the first few times you do it. Commit to trying something five times before trying something else. You'll be surprised what you end up enjoying.

WHY EXERCISE WORKS FOR WEIGHT LOSS BUT HAS LITTLE TO DO WITH BURNING CALORIES

If you walk on a treadmill for 30 min you are likely to burn about 100 calories.... very sad. Let's say you walk on that same treadmill 30 min every day for the next ten days! You will burn about 1000 calories. To put that in perspective 1 Caramel Frappuccino from Starbucks is 510 Calories, so 2 of those in 10 days and the 5 hrs or treadmill work was all for not! But if you walked for 30 minutes every day for ten days in a row you will lose weight and feel great.

So WHY does working out work?

First, when you exercise your body releases all kinds of endorphins and hormones and chemicals that trigger your brain and body to feel good. All those feelings of ecstasy do some great things.

- When you feel good, you make good decisions.
- When you make good decisions, you don't eat the junk.
- When you don't eat the junk, you save 100's or even 1000's of calories.

You may have burned 100 calories doing the exercise, but the feelings you get from exercise will save you from many more calories later. You will likely sleep better which means you'll have more energy in the morning and may not need that Caramel Frap to get you going like normal. You'll also be less likely to snack late at night.

Lastly, there is a carryover effect from exercise that adds together. You may have burned 100 calories during the activity, but your metabolism increases, and your body uses more calories repairing the damaged muscles. Also, stringing the same exercises together multiple days in a row will progress your ability. You'll be walking faster, and possibly even jogging by the end of the ten days so the first 30 min you burned 100 calories, the last 30 min you probably burned closer to 200.

There is a correlation between stored trapped fat and stored trapped emotions!

Science proves, exercising is a great tool for relieving stress and generating all those happiness chemicals. It's great for venting life frustrations, and I can't tell you how many times I've gone for a run, swim or bike ride and just screamed in my head to relieve emotional pressure.

It never fails, by the time my workout is finished, I have released emotions that were otherwise stuck. And when I'm on a good kick of exercising consistently the emotions have less time to pile up on top of each other. That translates into losing weight. One of my keys was learning that as I released my emotions and dealt with my fears and struggles that the weight just fell off of me.

We talked about the problem with cortisol and weight gain/ loss but here is where we get to take care of it. Cortisol is a product of stress so that we can effectively escape the danger that is in front of us. Since we mostly don't have to deal with a man-eating tiger in the cubicle next to us the release of that cortisol just doesn't happen, and it starts to pile up. Exercise is how you release cortisol.

All of your frustrations and problems can be worked out with exercise. If you have trouble smiling, getting a solid sweat going is an excellent way to get the corners of your mouth to curve upwards. No only are you releasing endorphins, serotonin, dopamine and a whole host of good vibes; you're also burning up that leftover cortisol.

So the benefits of exercising are many but know this. When you do get out there and start sweating, you'll make better decisions, smile more, sleep better, and be more fun to be around. If you're a guy, it helps with erectile dysfunction. In general, it also boosts sex drive for both men and women, so it helps marriages as well. If you want to double up on the relationship building aspect of it, then do an exercise together and get that Oxytocin going at the same time.

EXERCISE IS A NEED, BUT HOW TO DO IT EFFECTIVELY IS THE QUESTION?

In previous chapters we I talked about body types and body shapes. When it comes to exercise, they can be very helpful when maximizing your time. If you're like me and you're a mesomorph rectangle then pretty much everything you do will be effective except for abs. I'll probably never have that chiseled ab look. I'm not saying that it's not possible because there are abs of steel under the soft layer. If we did body sculpting workouts, they would show up. But it's more work for someone who is a triangle or hourglass shape.

I bring this up for an important reason; you will always look like you. If you get heavy into bodybuilding, then you'll look like the other body builders simply because of the extreme nature of that sport. If you plan on looking like a ballet dancer, then you better be an ectomorph body type, or you just won't ever look like that. It's time to detach from the outcome of our efforts and be happy with who we are, just as we are. Do exercises that help based on your body type and style, but ultimately you have to accept your biology.

BODY TYPES & HELPFUL EXERCISES

Ectomorph: Thin body, difficult to gain any muscle mass but great at losing weight. You will be most effective at endurance sports and exercises. If you're trying to lose weight, you'll be most effective running and other endurance sports. You will probably find that you enjoy the "runner's high" and will likely be ideal for cycling.

If you were thin for most of your life then "suddenly" gained a bunch of weight that you can't get off then most of the time you need to reset your metabolism. Focus on eliminating all refined sugar from your life and exercise back to back. Meaning if you only have time to exercise 2 days per week make them Saturday and Sunday or whatever two days you have available.

If you want to do weight lifting, there is no difference between you and someone else regarding potential strength, but it will be easier for others to gain muscle mass than you. Enjoy being the classic 50's movie star body type.

Mesomorph: Most of you are this body type, and is the classic "athletic style." You gain muscle mass easily and gain and lose weight quickly as well. You have an advantage in that anything you choose to do will be equally effective. Running and long distance sports will be more challenging in the beginning but will become easier and easier. Doing sport as a form of exercise will be very rewarding.

You won't lose weight as quickly as the ectomorph, but your muscle mass will show through faster. Your mantra should be calories in vs. calories out. Focus on consuming less food at each meal and eliminate the extra snacking and concentrate on doing little things throughout the day to keep your metabolism going like parking at the back of the parking lot or using the stairs instead of the elevator. The little things will add up and aid in your more intentional exercise program.

Approximately 70 percent of Americans are mesomorphs, so most of you are in this boat. Enjoy your natural ability to gain and lose mass.

Endomorph: Typically stocky but not always. You gain muscle mass very quickly and you're naturally strong. Your quickest path to fitness will be through strength exercises. Weightlifting, functional strength programs, and core strength exercises will yield the highest return. Don't discount running and general fitness exercise; it's a great way to balance out the strength.

If you're trying to "thin out" then focus on low weight and high repetition exercise. Running will help with being thinner and you may benefit from a "Fartlek" style approach which is something like run for 1 mile then walk for ½ mile then run another mile and walk another half mile and so on. Because you are strong, working on hills or stairs will be very rewarding, but it will also add mass to your legs.

I feel the need to encourage you endomorphs, because

you're body is great at holding onto mass it can be discouraging if you don't "look" thin. Enjoy the benefits of being strong and your ability to be fit.

QUICK EXERCISES

60/60 - Every 60 minutes do an exercise for 60 seconds and string this together 5-8 times per day five days in a row. Push-ups, Sit-ups/Crunches, Squats, Planks, Burpee's and Lunges are all great exercises that you can do anywhere even at work.

JOGGING - Head out your front door and go for a quick 20-30 min jog. It's easy and doesn't require anything more than a good pair of shoes. It's also something you can do during a lunch break, or if you are in a high-stress environment, it's an excellent way to end your work day before heading home. It doesn't have to be high intensity but doing it every day will help you a ton.

STRETCHING BREAK - Yoga is popular these days, but any general purpose stretching is great for you. It's quick easy and can be done anywhere without any equipment. Spend 15-30 minutes stretching and breathing. It's ideal for every exercise that you do to be limber, and it promotes blood flow to all parts of your body and clears cortisol. I like to end my day watching a little something on TV and stretching at the same time.

JUMP ROPE - Yes, and old fashioned jump rope is a great full body exercise, and you can do it in as little as 10 minutes per day. Also, it makes you feel kind of like a kid, so there's the added "fun" bonus. Jumping exercises, in general, are fantastic for your body.

TRAMPOLINE - Take a little trip on the trampoline, and you'll be amazed at the amount of fitness it takes to jump for 15-30 minutes. Some companies have built their entire business on trampoline fitness. You don't have to have a huge backyard bouncer; just a small personal trampoline is great. They range in price from $25 up to hundreds so just take a look at the weight specs and think about the amount of jumping you may do on it.

These are just a few of many quick exercises you can do just about anywhere. It's important that you find things to do that are fun and rewarding. Start a program at work where a group of you all do the 60/60 program. Your productivity will go way up as well. It helps you focus and keeps you feeling great.

Try creating a competition with a few friends and see how many days in a row you can jog without missing a day. Or see who can jump rope the most without messing up. Friendly group competitions are an excellent way to keep you motivated and also have fun.

None of these exercises will be fun at first, but the more you workout, the better you will feel and the more you'll enjoy it. I went for one year straight five days per week doing 300 push-ups per day because we all did this together in the office every day. Find a class at your local gym or a walking meet-up group. I've seen hiking groups at church and even kayaking groups. Joining other people having fun will be more fun and keep you involved. It's a great way to start.

EXERCISING & MUSIC

Avoid listening to music while training because it's transformational to be stuck with just your thoughts. I have found that having my mind full of the daily stresses, and internal struggles of wanting to quit before the first mile is an excellent way to train both my body and my mind. There's really nothing more healing than dealing with the things that are swirling around your head.

Avoid REPLAY - Be very cautious replaying events over and over in your head. You will begin to twist the facts and build emotions that never existed. If an event from the previous day or week comes up while exercising use your time as a way to let it go. If you need to forgive someone, then do it. If you need to yell and scream then do it. Don't stuff your stuff! Let it all out right now.

If you enjoy music and it's more fun to use it, then go for it! It's also a good time to listen to podcasts or books on tape and get some learning in at the same time, so it's not a hard and fast rule. Either way, deal with the emotions that show up and enjoy your time exercising.

DEALING WITH INJURY

Everyone deals with injuries on some level, so don't let that derail your fun. If you pull a muscle in your leg, then rest it. Do some upper body workouts instead. I know people in wheelchairs that exercise every day. Obviously, they aren't going for a run, but I've cycled with folks that use those hand cycles so don't let excuses keep you from enjoying life.

While playing soccer I've sprained my ankles and pulled hamstrings and other muscles but I never let it slow me down. I would strap up and keep playing anyway. I know this isn't the best advice medically so If you find yourself injured, it's important that you heal up as quickly as possible. For me, I have so much fun that I would rather limp down the field than not play. You may find that this is the case for you as well. Be sure you are doing the proper rehab and support to get better. Follow the advice of your doctor, because sometimes it's worth resting in the long run. I have often taken breaks from an activity I enjoy to make sure that I'm fully healed to get back to it.

If you get injured, don't stop exercising! Don't let it be an excuse to quit, but let it be an excuse to find something else fun to do while you're healing up. My friend loves to surf but once shattered his collarbone so he couldn't paddle through the waves. For rehab, he would do some stand-up paddle and light swimming instead. Eventually, he got back to his first love of surfing, but in the process, he found other fun things to do.

Recurring Injury -   If you have a recurring injury that stops you from having fun then see if it's something caused by what you're doing or if it's something deeper. I struggled with back pain for a long time. If I played basketball, I would likely pay for it later. I found out from Dr. Sarno and his book Healing Back Pain that my recurring back pain was an emotional attack that my mind was doing to my body because of financial stress. He wrote a whole book on the subject, so if you deal with that or any other recurring injury, then I recommend you read the book.

Nagging Injury - It's common to get a nagging injury that isn't enough to stop you from doing that thing you love but is sufficient to make it painful after. Fix it! If you're struggling with shin splints, plantar fasciitis or a nagging hamstring strain, it can stifle your fun. Some of these injuries are resolved with getting better shoes or some inserts. Sometimes, a simple ace bandage wrap can give enough support to heal up. Whatever it is, take care of it. Don't just let it keep nagging at you.

Preventative Injury - This is the most demoralizing to have an injury that prevents you from doing that one exercise you love to do. If it's something you can rehab and get back to your passion then take the time to do it. If it's something like a blown knee, then it's time to find something else to enjoy. Don't dwell on your loss but find something else fun. I love playing soccer, but I also love swimming, and I discovered that cycling is a great exercise. Always accentuate the positives and ignore the negatives. You may find a brief grieving period where you feel a loss from what you love to do, but there are lots of amazing fun things in the world.

EXERCISE PROGRAM

Regardless of what program you decide to try, find something that you have fun doing. Some people love extreme exercise like the P90X, and others prefer to relax and yoga it up. There is no right or wrong way to get out and exercise. The benefit of exercising far outweighs the calorie burning aspect, so the intensity only impacts the speed at which you lose weight.

The idea behind the *Fun Diet* is to enjoy your life. A 90-day program isn't the lifelong answer; it's a process. You're simply doing things that add to your overall enjoyment and will ultimately help keep you fit and feeling great for the rest of your life. The *Fun Diet* is a lifestyle change and a mental shift, not a one-time solution.

Do the 30-day programs and take the 7-day challenges. Have fun trying out different group programs and sports. In the process discover the things inside that are keeping you stuck and deal with them. Use the exercise as a way to build your mental strength as well. When the task is hard like training for your first Mud Race or Half Marathon, use that time to help be successful in other areas of your life as well.

We were made for challenges. Our bodies were designed for physical activity and when we ignore that then our bodies start to give up. Now is your time, go get it!

THINGS I'VE MISSED OUT ON IN THE PAST BECAUSE OF MY HEALTH OR WEIGHT

_____

_____

_____

_____

_____

_____

_____

_____

_____

_____

_____

_____

_____

_____

Chapter 8
30 DAY **BE** TRAINNG

Identity is half of the equation when it comes
to breakthrough. Getting this right is key to a
lifetime of healthy weight.

The first part of The Fun Diet is getting your "BE" working for you. The BE is your identity and is the most important part of having a lifetime of healthy weight. When stuck in any part of life the main issue is our Belief System; I call our BS. We have developed half truths and false thinking around those areas. The BS we use will create the lens for how we act, react, and plan that part of our life. With unhealthy weight patterns and food related issues, one of the biggest areas that I work on is the things we say to ourselves in the mirror, both literally and figuratively.

Take the next 30 Days to find the core of who you are in this area of your life. I keep saying "this area of your life" because it's very common for people to be very successful in other parts of life without having success in all of them. Oprah is a good example of this. We can all agree that she is a wildly successful businesswoman and media mogul. She has been very successful at what we see from her publicly. However, in interviews, she admits that her struggle with weight is the last mountain that she wants to conquer.

Being stuck here doesn't mean anything about the rest of your life. We are going to work specifically on getting your BS to serve you instead of taking you down. It's time to take control of the thoughts in your head, the identity in your heart, and lens that see yourself through.

WEEK 1: PREPARE
You Are Not What You Eat, You Are WHY You Eat

Our WHY is very powerful. If you think about a mother protecting her child, her WHY will cause her to do anything regardless of rationale to save that child. For example, if someone were to threaten her child's life she will give her own up without blinking to save the child's. Why we go to work every day isn't to make money, it's to have the security we need to feed ourselves and family and keep a roof over our head. Why we eat isn't because we are hungry and need fuel. There are many times we eat even when we're not hungry, and there are many times that we've technically eaten enough and yet we're still hungry.

Finding our WHY brings freedom and breakthrough. What are we after? Freedom from the weight battle and breakthrough from the struggle.

PREPARE

This week is preparation week. We need to prepare to go on this journey. In preparation for our victory we need to ask ourselves, "WHY?" Keep a journal if you would like, or just make notes on your smartphone. Every time you eat something or decide NOT to eat something ask yourself "Why?"

- What you are eating isn't as important as why you're eating (or not eating). I say "Or not eating" because a very high percent of people who have food issues don't eat breakfast.

- Ask yourself WHY when you decide on something like diet soda vs. regular or super-sizing vs. having the normal meal or going back for seconds or in my case thirds.

Don't second guess yourself and do something different than your routine unless it's an obvious poor choice. I want you to continue to do what you have always done. This week is not about changing anything. We need just to be conscious about why so next week we can start getting into the bigger questions and do the real work.

EXAMPLES

- I chose diet soda over water because I need my soda.
- I chose diet soda because I don't want the calories that sugar has.
- I picked the Big Mac because it's convenient and cheap.
- I supersized the meal because they asked me if I wanted to and it sounded good.
- I didn't eat breakfast because I don't have time.
- I didn't eat breakfast because it makes my stomach hurt.
- I ate dessert because it was being offered to me and I don't want to offend.
- I chose cookies because I deserve a little something.
- I'm eating because I'm bored.

Dig deeper and ask second and third questions to get to the root.

I'm eating this bag of chips because I'm hungry and it's convenient and quick to eat. I'm hungry because it's midnight and I ate dinner at 6pm, and it's time to eat again. I'm up this late because I deserve a break and need my alone time. I need my alone time because the kids are overwhelming me and I can't seem to get a break when they're awake.

Be thoughtful about your "Whys." Take time to think through "why." "Because I'm hungry" is an obvious why, but doesn't explain about the food that you chose. Go deep here; it's time to get truly honest with yourself about why you're eating a fourth meal or not eating breakfast. If it's been 4 hours since your last meal then you will be hungry, but why are you up that late? Is it stress, fear, boredom, anxiety? I used to stay up late because I was trying to take more time before the next day showed up and I had to go to work. Be thoughtful of your answers.

THIS WEEK

1. Keep track of why you are eating the things that you are. Be conscious of your choices. We will be grouping them together next week and using them to start succeeding. Do this five days this week.

2. Start to think about the true WHY's in your life that will keep you going when things get tough. If you've ever been on a diet before then, you know that it brings up a lot of emotions, self-doubt, and struggle. We are going to combat those ahead of time. Think about why you want to lose weight? Why does it

matter that you slay the weight demon once and for all? Why do you want to be free from the shame and struggle of being overweight?

3. Be thoughtful about your answers. This is your opportunity to dig deep and find out what is truly holding you back. If you need some help with this, join our private Facebook group and post your why there and ask for help. I'll be checking in on it, and other people will be supporting your journey. -

facebook.com/groups/fundiet

4. Week 1 is preparation week, so I truly don't want you changing anything. What I do want, is for you to reflect on what you want to get out of this. Plan on this being the last program you will ever need for your weight loss journey. Every day for 7 days when you wake up tell yourself that this is your time to win. There is no hurry to lose weight, and there are no requirements for what needs to happen. Your goal is a lifetime of healthy weight so if it takes a little time to start seeing the effects of your changes then so be it. Plan on making one good decision at a time and know that your breakthrough will come from inside and not what you're eating.

WEEK 2: REFRAME
Powerful or Powerless

Look at your notes from last week to why or why not and start to gather them into as few themes as possible. A theme is where you see a similar type of why.

SOME EXAMPLES:

- I chose diet soda over water because I need my soda. - I need

- I chose diet soda because I don't want the calories that sugar has. - Saving Calories

- I didn't eat breakfast because I don't have time. - I don't have time

- I didn't eat breakfast because it makes my stomach hurt. - I don't like the way I feel

- I chose cookies because I deserve a little something. - I deserve

EXAMPLE THEMES:

- Convenient
- Boredom
- I Deserve
- I Don't Want
- Saving Calories
- I Don't Like The Way I Feel When
- My Doctor Suggested
- I Just Like This
- You Aren't Taking My
- I always

There are no hard and fast themes, just group your "Whys." Develop a few that make sense. If it's more than three, then that's ok as well. Maybe you will get 6 or 8 then try to narrow them down more if possible.

The main purpose for this week is to reframe your thinking.

The decisions you're making about food are conscious. Maybe they are right choices, and your reasons for them are strong. If they are bad decisions then why are you making them? Is it lack of training or information. Is it because you feel you are missing something.

Is it fear? Fear of gaining weight, being a failure, proving everyone who has ever mocked you right, etcetera. Fear, shame, and doubt, all kind of fall into the same category, and are one of the main causes of doing things that are bad for us. When fear creeps in, we do irrational things and have trouble discerning better options than our default decision.

Is it stress? Stress could be more than just pressure it can be not acknowledging feelings or even anxiety. Don't discount stress. A lot of our WHY's can be bunched into the Stress eating category. Often, when I have been working real hard or feel like I'm being under-appreciated, I will REWARD myself with a treat.

What starts as one treat might end up in weeks of treats. I discovered that once I "fell off the wagon" so to speak then I would continue making bad food decisions. It's important that you realize there is no wagon. You're not on a restrictive diet; you are on a fun diet, and you need to enjoy your life in the process.

> **The solution:** Acknowledge that I need a treat. Ask why. Realize that it's because I am feeling under-appreciated. Then make a good decision. If I still want the treat, then I will get it and eat it. I still need to address why I'm feeling under-appreciated. It can be as simple as talking with my spouse about how I'm feeling. You may need to speak with your boss or someone else. Or you could work out why you're feeling that way on your own and resolve it. The key here is that you address the emotion. Talking it out or even writing about it are great ways to process the emotion completely. I prefer to deal with my emotions while exercising, then talk through what's going on with my wife after.

Once you identify the why, and make the decision to have the treat or not, you will not end in spiraling out of control for weeks at a time. Own the decision to satisfy your feelings with the food. Then plan on making a better decision next time. Identifying the WHY isn't about feeling shame, it's about empowering yourself to succeed.

THIS WEEK

STEP 1 - Continue to ask why you're making the food choices that you are, but this week decide to change whether you do or don't, based on your internal dialog.

STEP 2 - Change everything. (Don't worry, it's only for this week)

Breakfast - If you don't eat breakfast regularly make sure you eat something within the first hour of you being awake. If you do eat breakfast, I want you to change what you usually eat with something very different. If it's cereal then have an egg, if it's an egg have cereal (nothing sugary, try to eat something that won't kill you). You can choose to do a smoothie or juice carrots or something not too fruity.

BREAKFAST IDEAS:

Morning juice recipe - 8-12 carrots & 1 Grapefruit (peeled). If buying juice from the market, stay away from fruit heavy juices and no smoothies. It's about nutrition, and I want you to get extra doses of veggies. Suja is a good brand of regular market available juices.

Morning smoothie - ½ cup oats, 1 banana, 2 tablespoons hemp seeds, 1 tablespoon chia seeds, 1 handful of almonds, water or milk for desired thickness.

Morning cereal - Old Fashioned Rolled Oats - Fruit (banana, raisins, or seasonal fruit) - Cinnamon - Splash of Honey

Morning egg breakfast - 2 eggs, 2 handfuls of spinach, chopped green onions. 1 piece of toast.

LUNCH - Pack a lunch if you can. If you can't do that, then change where and what you eat. The point of this is to change everything. It's only for the week so do your best. If you always get a burger, then find a place to get a salad or a taco or anything other than your norm.

Start trying to make better decisions about the food you're eating. This is an excellent opportunity to go to that crazy health food store and get a strange wrap. Packing a lunch is the best option.

DINNER - Change it up. Whatever you usually eat, do something different. NO EATING OUT. Watch a video if you have to. Try something new that you've never had before. Make a plan for the week and go shopping now so there are no excuses. Plan a "quick" dinner for that day you might be rushed for time. Try not to make anything for 7 days that you normally make. Go crazy with it and have some fun!

4TH MEAL - For many eating late at night is a struggle, mostly because you're awake. Go to bed! I understand how it is though and I often still enjoy a late night snack. For this week and until you can get better habits and technique don't eat the fourth meal. If you're "starving" then have a warm liquid (caffeine free). A hot herbal tea satisfies, or even a warm glass of milk is a fun treat and will help you go to sleep.

BONUS: Stay away from 'Skim' or 'Low-Fat' milk, if you're going to have milk make it "whole" milk. Those others are not nearly as satisfying and the fat is where all the nutrition is.

WEEK 3 - CREATE
Am I Acceptable?

A question that everyone faces regardless of weight is, "Am I Acceptable?". It's an issue that humanity has struggled with forever. At some point, you will wonder if you are good enough, have what it takes, or if you are even lovable.

Your emotions are a mash of chemical reactions, hormones, sensory input, and memories. A lot of what we "feel" can be a direct result of a belief system (BS) that we developed at a young age. So, think about the 8-year-old version of yourself and A you trust that version to make your current list of life choices? Would you trust them to plan your meals or budget your household or give you relationship advice? The answer is of course not.

A lot of what we do now is based on beliefs and decisions we made when younger. A lot of what holds us back and keeps us stuck is based on things that happened to us and not choices that we've made. Many people get stuck before they ever have a chance to find out for themselves.

STORY TIME:

I was playing basketball at my local gym, and I blocked this guy's shot well. The whole gym shouted their pleasure with my accomplishment. Now, this guy was obviously embarrassed and to be honest he was one of the better players on the court. You could say I got lucky. I wouldn't say that but someone else might :)

Play continues and without warning he runs into me, in the back. I used to play football, so I didn't think much of it. The next play he does it again, then again. Then I have an opportunity to stand in front of him (called setting a pick) and let him crash into me. Once again he goes flopping to the floor rejected. He instantly pops up and wants to fight.

> My response was, "What are we doing? Are we going to fist fight like children? Let's have fun!"

> After a brief, tense moment, we ended up shaking hands and getting back to play.

His decisions were not made from the place of adult critical thinking. He wanted to prove he was tougher (even though I was much larger & stronger). That was not the decision of a grown man. It came from a place that started when he was younger and probably has something to do how he was raised.

How many times in our lives do we listen to the young version of ourselves who was abandoned, rejected, abused, hurt, laughed at, mistreated, and ignored?

It's time to develop a new Belief System.

I AM ACCEPTABLE

My wife chose me and accepts me. My kids accept me, flaws and all. My clients accept me. My family and friends accept me. All that was left was ME. Could I accept me?

Some of you may not have a similar support system that I do, but if you look hard enough, there are people that accept you. If you've ever been hired for a job or accepted into a school, then you have been accepted. But let's take it one step further. Does any of that matter? There is only one person in the world whose opinion matters. Yours!

If you don't feel acceptable, it's because you don't accept yourself. Why is entirely up to you to figure out from your own journey. If you struggle with this, it's because there is a young version of you that told you how to judge your life.

It's time to create a grown-up perspective. Your actions and decisions can be judged as acceptable or not acceptable, and you have control over those. But you at your core cannot be judged as acceptable or not. YOU ARE ACCEPTABLE just as you are at your core. Learning how to react well, and interact with others well is a learned skill and behavior. We do many things out of habit or because we have fear or shame about them. A good book about this is *Daring Greatly* - by Brené Brown.

This Week
IT'S PERSPECTIVE TIME!

3 Times Every Day look into a mirror or a reflection of yourself and say the opposite of whatever it is with which you struggle. This is not a cheesy trick. You are creating a new lens.

- I AM ACCEPTABLE
- I AM LOVABLE, AND I AM LOVED
- I DO HAVE WHAT IT TAKES
- I AM GOOD ENOUGH

Do this Several Times when you're getting ready for your day, in the middle of the day, and before you go to bed. Try to repeat this

10 times at minimum every day this week. These are just samples to get you started. Find your own areas of struggle and say the opposite to yourself. Try to find a minimum of 3 and a maximum of 5 for this week. After that, do whatever you want.

NOTE: Some of my clients who struggle with depression have a real problem with this exercise at first. It can actually cause them to get worse not better. The way out has been to understand that the purpose isn't some positivity woo woo training but that this is how to reprogram your neural pathways.

TRUTH

The truth is not relative, it simply is. A glass of water filled half way is both half full and half empty. Those are conditions. The truth is that it contains 4 oz of water and 4 oz of air. Stating a positive condition doesn't change the truth, just the state of being. When you use truth to state an opposite condition it isn't changing the truth, just aligning with a different state of being.

The truth is that you are acceptable just as you are. If you never lose any weight and are "heavy" for the rest of your life, it only affects how you feel and fit into clothing. You are the same person thick or thin.

Ultimately you will need to accept yourself. You don't have to accept things that you can change like your weight or your clothing; but you will have to accept things that you can't change, like your height or where you were born and who you were born to. You can't change your past, and you can't change how others act towards you, but what you can change is your future and how you act and react.

Your future is your own and if you want it to be different, then now is the time to start making changes. Enjoy the process and find a way to accept yourself just as you are.

WEEK 4 - SUCCESS
Practice Positivity

A friend of mine says, "Whatever is acceptable will become inevitable." I couldn't agree with that statement more. If your pants are getting too tight and you go out and buy a pair that fits better you have accepted the new size, and you will soon fill those pants out completely as well.

I'm not saying that it's a bad idea to feel comfortable in the clothes that you're wearing but I am saying that feeling uncomfortable isn't always a bad thing, especially if we are using it as a tool for change.

I'm a waist size 36. Most of the time those are a bit loose on me, but I don't fit in size 34 and thinking I will fit in them is probably not intelligent. I'm 6'2" and I would have to lose a bunch of muscle mass to do that. The big BUT, no pun intended, is that I have purchased pants that are 38, and 40, and higher. It has never served me. It was a temporary shift to feel comfortable and look right in my clothing. The reality is, if sitting in my size 36 pants all day like a stuffed sausage is a problem for me, then I am more likely to think about eating that donut in the break-room. Ok, this section isn't about clothing, it's just an example.

What I want to talk about is what things in your life have you accepted as true about you? We've gone over this before a bit. Maybe it's something like, "I will always be bigger." Or, "I'm too old to lose the weight." How about, "What's the point, I'm just going to gain it back anyway."

Self defeating prophecies will ALWAYS come true.

If you say you are bad at something, more than likely you will prove yourself correct the next time you attempt it. The good news is that this also works in the positive direction. The more you talk, act, and think about the "cans" instead of the "can't-s" the better the outcome will be for you.

This Week

Think about the areas of your life that you accept negative thoughts, words, and actions as the way they will always be. Write them down, then re-write how they should be. Once you start treating yourself properly, then other people will follow suit.

Write some positive self-fulfilling prophecies. Start writing about how you will look and feel in the future. Write down positive replacement statements for your negative one.

Even something as normal as "Losing Weight" is a negative even though it represents something positive. A positive statement is, "I'm getting down to a healthy weight." Start correcting yourself when you hear the negative statement. Practice positivity.

Keep notes and when you think a negative thought about yourself, or say it out loud, or if someone else says it to you and it hurts, then write those things down. Later when you have time, reframe those into a positive way. It's time to reject the negative self-talk once and for all.

NOTES

NOTES

NOTES

Chapter 9
30 DAY **FEEL** TRAINNG

Are you living your life or is your life living you?

WEEK 1: PREPARE
Personal Responsibility

One of the greatest deceptions about diets and exercises is that we are dependent on them for our success. IF we don't lose weight or even if we do lose weight but it didn't give us permanent results, then IT didn't work. You don't need anything in this book to be successful if you own the responsibility for how you look and feel. You will either find contentment where you're currently at or make a change. **Taking personal responsibility for the outcome of our life releases our superpower for change.**

It's easy to believe things that are self-defeating and keep us from achieving our goals even before we ever start.

BELIEF: It's genetic and is harder for me to lose weight than other people. Translation - I'm just different, and I will always be fat, I was born that way.

REALITY: If you put your own food in your own mouth then you are the master of your own fate. Regardless of body type or genetics at the end of the day, we are the ones that decide to eat the cookie and not workout.

There are specific techniques that we need to learn based on our body types, but if we believe that we are not capable of change, then there is no point to try.

BELIEF: I'm not a good athlete, and it's difficult for me to exercise. I end up hurting myself and then it's worse than before. Translation: I'm not good enough to do what other people can do; I will always fail.

REALITY: You don't need to be athletic to exercise. You don't need to do crazy training regimens to fit in. If you are not comfortable going to CrossFit for example, then walk around the block, or just lift weights the old fashioned way; or play some ultimate frisbee; or just go for a walk every day. There is always something you can be doing and if you decide to sit on the couch and watch TV instead it is your decision.

PERSONAL RESPONSIBILITY TIME

It is very important that we come to the belief that we are the designers of our fate. I say it all the time, "Are you living your life or is your life living you?" Are you the result of where you born, who you were born to, and what people have done to you? (I'll cheat and give you the answer - NOPE)

There are many people who we can use as examples that were born all wrong and grew up to do great things. You get to believe what you want. Your belief makes your reality. I'm NOT saying there is no such thing as absolutes, and I'm not giving you permission to abandon reason. I AM saying that PERSPECTIVE is one of the greatest tools in your tool belt.

You see once we take full responsibility for where we are in our life. We stop blaming Mom & Dad and our boss and that one kid in high school that messed up our life. Something magical happens. We are now FREE to create the world in which we want to live.

STORY

I have a good friend who was abused in every way possible. He was abandoned by both his parents and torn apart emotionally and physically by many awful people. He was suicidal and depressed and by the time he was 16 he had tried to commit suicide a dozen times. He grew up to be a successful entrepreneur and has an amazing life with a beautiful wife and kids. He took responsibility for his future and left the past where it belonged.

His story is not unique. It's rare because we learn to be defeated, but it's not unique. There are many others just like it.

HERE'S MY CHALLENGE TO YOU:

TAKE RESPONSIBILITY FOR YOUR FUTURE

From this day forward I am the master of my fate. I will not allow anything that I have been told, given, or expected, to stop me from my goals and to live my life to the fullest. I have chosen my current life, and if I don't like it, then I will make different choices.

THIS WEEK

The rest of this week you will take personal responsibility. I mean it. When some jack cuts you off in traffic, you will take responsibility for driving in your space. You didn't deserve their intrusion, and you are justified in being upset. HOWEVER, it will not serve you to be upset. Just because you have the right doesn't make it good for you.

You will say, "Wow they must be in a hurry." You will slow down and give them some space. And you will take responsibility for driving in your own space, and you will benefit from letting them get out of your life as quickly as they came into it. Do this for everything this week, including food and exercise choices.

If you are not exercising regularly or not eating healthy, it's time to take responsibility. I'm not asking you to change anything... yet... but I do want you to own your choices.

> **Blame Statement:** I am craving chocolate, and I have to eat it.

> **Changes to:** I have a need that chocolate is filling. I choose to eat the chocolate now and figure out why I'm craving it later. I'll discover tools to change this or accept it as something to enjoy.

> **Or this:** I am craving chocolate, and I choose not to fill that desire because my cravings don't control me.

Either one is good, just make it YOUR CHOICE!

WEEK 2: REFRAME
Powerful Self Talk

One of the things that I struggled with a lot was getting down on myself. The shame of making poor decisions or just looking in the mirror and saying horrible things was a part of my daily life. I would beat myself up then fill the emotional hole I just created, with food.

I ate very healthily, and we never kept junk food in the house, not to mention that we made almost everything from scratch. So WHY was I overweight.... simple... I ate a ton of food.

Organic cookies are still cookies. 3 Plates of healthy food for dinner is still three plates of food. The problem was not with what I was eating. It was why I was eating and why I couldn't STOP.

The truth is that I was setting myself up for failure. There were several times per day where I would think about my weight. I would look in the mirror and say negative defeating things. I would give myself excuses that no one could dispute.

Example:

I'm just a big guy, and I'm happy with my weight.

No one could dispute those two "facts." The truth is that I'm a tall guy at 6'2" and I used to bench press 500lbs. To do that I needed to have a very muscular large frame. Today, I'm not nearly as muscular. What changed? Nothing, I'm the same guy. The truth is I'm a tall guy. My size was just how I chose to look.

When I said, "I'm happy with my weight." That was not true either. The TRUTH is that I was ashamed. To be truly honest, I was unhappy with the way I looked despite what I used to say to other people. I would rationalize, and positive-think myself into believing that I was happy with it. The reality is that I was happy with ME but not the weight.

WHY DO I BRING ALL THIS UP?

There are many times throughout your day where you believe and speak back to yourself powerless thoughts and statements. STOP IT! You are worth more than that.

The fact that you bought this book is PROOF that you believe you are worth more than that. It's time to turn your powerless victim-based thinking into POWERFUL SELF TALK.

This Week:
Make A List

Make a list of the negative or powerless things that you say to yourself throughout the day.

Write down ANYTHING that relates to your genetics, where and who you were born to, your past, or any other situation that is outside of your control, stop speaking those things immediately.

You cannot do anything about your past, but you can do something about your future.

Where you are TODAY is a product of what you did YESTERDAY, so if you want to be somewhere different TOMORROW, then you have to OWN your choices NOW.

POWERFUL SELF TALK

1) If you think that you were born fat or born to be fat, change the perspective a bit and own where you are today. An example: I was born to an overweight family. Everyone in my family is overweight. I learned how to eat and treat myself from them. Apparently, they make poor choices. I will make good choices from this day forward. I was born for freedom, and being overweight doesn't feel free.

2) When you say something bad to yourself in the mirror, instantly flip it over. I would say things like this: "Looking good, fat ass! Did you enjoy the box of donuts last night!" ---- Instantly Say: "Don't talk about me that way. I am changing my life, and it takes practice. Looking good, just looking good.

This isn't a cheesy thing to do, it's real. The things you say to yourself and about yourself are real, and it works both ways. If you say negative defeating words, then you will feel defeated. If you say positive freeing words, then you will feel free.

How you feel, is how you will act.

3) During the day you may get comments about your weight, or even there may be consequences for being overweight like, you can't take the stairs or sit in that one chair. These are all external things that hurt us. You don't need to stick up for yourself, but what you need to do is OWN it.

> **Example 1:** Your friend is trying to be helpful and asks about your weight. They think they can help you lose weight because they are skinny. They say, "I'm your friend and I care about you. I know you've struggled with losing weight and I think I can help." INSTANTLY you may think... "You skinny little.... you have no idea what I've gone through and tried, there just isn't any hope for me. Now leave me alone!"

INSTEAD OWN IT - "I've struggled with weight in the past because I didn't believe in myself. I didn't have other people who believed in me, and I learned how to be bad to myself. As hard as I tried to lose weight in the past, it was stuck because I was stuck. Today I know that my choices are keeping me, stuck. I'm overweight because I just couldn't stop. Stop eating, stop hating, stop stuffing my emotions."

The difference in all of these examples is that you are taking ownership of your future.

> **Example 2:** You are going to a friends house, and they have one chair that you hope you don't have to sit in. It has cracked and creaked a lot, and you would be devastated if it broke while you were sitting on it. You feel fear and shame and maybe will make an excuse to leave if you have to sit in that

chair this time.

INSTEAD OWN IT - By this time next year, I will be sitting in that chair with confidence. Don't make an excuse, everyone in that room knows your situation, so you're not losing anything by being vulnerable. You can say, "Hey can sit in the big chair, I'm nervous about this one's survival if I sit in it. I'm working a program right now that is making me be vulnerable with you and this time next year I will proudly sit in that one, but today I want the big one."

I hope you hear my heart in this. There is FREEDOM in being honest and vulnerable with yourself. It is BRAVE to take the powerful position. Ultimately where you are tomorrow is based on what you do today. So today, get it!

WEEK 3: CREATE
Declarations of Acceptance

Don't let this sections scare you off. We're not talking about a mystical spiritual thing; it's simply a useful tool for conditioning your mind.

One of the things that you can count on is that your emotions play a vital role in the decisions that you make on a moment by moment basis. If you were bitten by a dog when you were little, there is a chance that all dogs regardless of size can cause you some anxiety.

The same applies to our behaviors in other areas. If we say negative powerless things to ourselves often enough, then we will act accordingly. It's not the other way around.

Saying that you will always be heavy will cause your body to say "ok" and join in on making it so. As we begin to make powerful statements in place of self-defeating ones, then the other areas of our life will line up with those statements.

Complaining about yourself and others or thinking that self-deprivation is humorous or criticizing people publicly is damaging to you and others. Comments that are coming out of our mouth automatically without any conscious thought about what is being said is called speaking unconsciously, and it must stop. Intentional speaking should replace it. We may need help from others to help us catch ourselves until new habits form. Discontinue as fast as possible cursing yourself and others and speak blessing instead.

Let's take for example the belief that you are genetically heavy and it's just too difficult to overcome genetics. First of all, if you didn't eat anything for the next 180 days, you would be emaciated. We can agree that your body would consume all the excess fats and muscles on your body and you would be skin and bones.

It is true that there are several body types. It is also true that how our families dealt with food, nutrition, and body image impacted and continues to affect how we eat now. We believe that we are STUCK, and so we are stuck.

I have seen where one person in a family breaks free and loses a bunch of weight then slowly others in the same family follow suit. What happened? The other people saw that it was possible and they made powerful statements like, "If my sister can do it, then I can do it too."

Here are some common curses:

- I'm so tired
- I am addicted to sweets
- I have always been big
- I can't lose weight, I've tried
- It is just the way I am, etcetera.

When you speak negative unloving words repeatedly, you are making that which you don't want to be your reality.Blessing yourself is making statements of truth about yourself as you want to be and results you want in your life.

This weeks mindset challenge will be to reverse your powerless talk into how you want to see yourself in the future. The goal here is to be bold and make a crazy dream. You don't have to believe that it's possible to achieve the dream; just dream.

Make them current, not future tense: I am... I look... I feel....

Here are a few to get you started:

- I am making positive changes, and my life is getting better every day.
- I take good care of myself because I am worth it.
- God made me unique, and I love myself just the way I am.
- I am a perfect weight.
- I am free from the struggle with weight once and for all.

THIS WEEK

Make a list of declarations and decrees and put copies in your car, bathroom, desk and any place else you can see them, so you can read your declarations repeatedly during the day. The more often you speak these blessings over yourself, family, home and work the sooner they will be your reality.

1. Write them out on note cards; dry erase boards, lipstick on the bathroom mirror, reminders on your smartphone.

2. Write them, re-write them, speak them out loud, read them to yourself and share them with others.

3. If you find 1 or 2 declarations to be particularly useful, then share them with our Facebook group.

WEEK 4: SUCCESS
Have Fun

One of the greatest aha moments of my life was when I discovered how to have fun. It was when I learned how to enjoy the process of life that I was free to be me.

A life lesson about mindset is that the lens that you CHOOSE to see your life, family, health, and work through will impact your overall success in that area. You CAN change your perspective, and in doing so, you will change your outcome.

Successful weight loss is not about dropping the pounds, but in never struggling with it again. Having a proper mindset is what makes the struggle disappear.

Diets are restrictive and annoying or worse yet; they are not even healthy for you. Enjoying what you're eating and cooking will make sustaining a healthy lifestyle possible. If you are getting good feedback from your family and the people who are supporting you, then you are more likely to continue. Being part of a group of people all facing the same challenges will make you 35% more likely to be successful.

The message for this week is to Have Fun with whatever "technique" you are using to lose weight. Even just deciding only to do and eat things that you enjoy is a good test for this week. If you enjoy eating a pint of ice cream at midnight, then you should probably edit that decision. Honestly, it's not fun to be overweight. It's not fun to feel like crap, and it's not fun to know that you are not doing the right things.

Choose to be healthy, choose to see the amazing qualities of healthy food, and learn to enjoy eating them.

This Week

Find a meal each day this week that you can eat and you enjoy! Make sure it's not McD's fast food or something that is killing you. If it's a burger, then grill up a high-quality-meat burger, and get some good ingredients to go on top of it. If your diet plan doesn't allow certain foods, then find some things that you can do which are enjoyable and plan those for one meal each day this week.

Journal about what the joy is with that meal, and learn what "NEED" is that food fulfilling. It could be something as simple as, "my mom always made this soup, and I need comfort." Then you know that the food isn't the need, "Comfort" is the need. Then you can fulfill the actual need instead of medicating with massive quantities of bad-for-you food.

Begin to fill your "NEED" with something other than food. Most of the time it will be only one or two different common themes that cause overeating or medicating with food.

JOURNAL

_____

_____

_____

_____

_____

_____

_____

_____

_____

_____

JOURNAL

JOURNAL

Chapter 10

30 DAY **DO** TRAINNG

Do the right techniques with a proper mindset and a true identity and you **will** be successful.

Technique is all about supporting our natural abilities and talents; or overcoming deficiencies. It's important that we are serious about learning how to eat healthy and be healthy. The quality of our health significantly impacts the quality of our life. If you "can't" participate in fun things in your life it will cause you to spiral downward in your weight journey.

Many people don't "like" health food or vegetables. It's time to grow up. No one liked coffee the first time they drank it, and many foods are not great if the only exposure to them are low-quality versions. All real food is great! Did you know that your taste buds are 100% new every week? That means that the food you like can change within a week.

Exercise is all about technique. If you do an exercise, incorrectly it may not be as fun or effective, and you could hurt yourself. Taking your time to learn how to be active properly is wise. Having said that, if you don't just try things and make a mess of them, then you may never learn how to do something that you may ultimately love.

Above all, enjoy the process of becoming healthy. You may discover after a couple of weeks you're looking forward to exercising. And after successfully eating healthy for a bit you may find that you enjoy feeling better and will want to continue.

WEEK 1 PREPARE
Simple Changes To Setup Your Success

Often the difference between success and failure is something small. I've found that taking one week to prepare to make crazy changes is the best way to form a pattern interrupt and get the best results. This week we are going to keep it super simple and just set up next week's success.

EXERCISE

Plan your exercise program for the next week. Do your research and if you're looking for groups to join or places to play a sport find them this week and the times. Put it on your calendar for next week if you need to, but make your plans now. Also, make sure you take it slow. If you haven't already been exercising, don't plan something challenging to do every day.

I recommend that you pick two things to try next week that will be 1-2 hours of moderate exercise. If you're going to do some intense training, then keep the time shorter. You want to have fun and enjoy yourself.

DIET

This week we aren't changing too much, just a few tricks to start you off right.

One and Done - This is an easy way to keep from overeating. No seconds, just have one plate of food.

If you're eating fast food, which obviously is not a good idea only chose one item. No "Meals" and no multiple items off the dollar menu. Pick one and be done.

Eat Breakfast - If you usually don't eat breakfast, this week and for the rest of your life, you will now eat breakfast. It is the most important meal of the day. Don't eat junk food and sugary stuff for breakfast. A donut is NOT breakfast. Breakfast should be a balanced meal that sets up the rest of your day. A small bowl of cereal that is low on sugar like unsweetened shredded wheat or some rolled oats with a pinch of honey are a great option. Muesli is a healthy breakfast that you can eat cold with milk or hot with water. Don't worry about fruit sugar, fresh fruit is great for you and is good at breakfast, but avoid as much refined sugar as possible.

Some people do better on protein in the morning, so eggs are a good option. There are lots of ways to cook eggs, but if you can add some greens to them, it's a good idea.

If you find it difficult to eat breakfast, then go for a piece of toast and ½ grapefruit; or something else light. The idea is to start your metabolism firing within 1 hour of waking up.

Hot Liquid - Having some hot liquid instead of snacking is a great way to give your body and gut a break from digesting food. It also satiates hunger and if you're drinking herbal options they generally have other significant health benefits. If you're

trying to avoid eating late at night, some warm milk
is good.

Next week you will be juicing. Read ahead to next week and decide
if you're going to use a juicer or buy pre-made juice; either way, no
blenders. I love smoothies, but the idea isn't to have one carrot and
a bunch of water but to have a dozen carrots or 2 whole bunches
of greens, etc. It's all about adding nutrition, not fiber. You can get
fiber in other ways if you need it, which you probably don't for one
week.

**This week is preparation and is all about setting yourself up to
have success and fun.**

WEEK 2: REFRAME
Juicing Breakfast
& New Exercises

Juicing was one of the biggest helps on my journey.

One of the benefits of juicing is to supercharge your nutrition. Often
you are hungry throughout the day only because you aren't eating
food rich in nutrition and although you are getting the calories,

your body isn't getting all the other nutrients that it needs.

If you want to do what I did then, you will buy a juicer and a bunch of carrots, grapefruit, kale, spinach, apples, lemons, & ginger.

I juiced carrots and grapefruit for breakfast (warning grapefruit will counteract medicine so if you are taking medication juice an orange instead with your carrots.) Then I would pre-juice and bottle with me for lunch the Kale, Spinach, 1 apple, 1 lemon, 1-inch ginger.

Later I would eat a sensible dinner. I also stayed away from all sweets during this week.

If that is too hardcore for you, try just replacing your breakfast with juiced carrots. Don't get a big bottle from the shelf; it must be from the refrigerated section with an expiration date and nothing added to it. Not from concentrate, and no added sugar or water. Just straight up juiced vegetables. Stay away from all fruit juices, and focus on the ones with mostly vegetables in them. If for health reasons you can't replace breakfast with juice, then add juice to your breakfast routine.

Food is your friend, not your enemy. Use it to fuel your life and help you get good results.

This Week

Eat your breakfast or drink your juice within 1 hour of waking up. If you're doing the juice thing like I did, then this is your week to feel the power of juice. Don't use a blender; that is not the kind of juicing I'm referring. You can always get your fiber in the rest of your meals, but for 7 days in a row you will be juicing 8-15 carrots for breakfast (Or other vegetables of your choosing).

> **Morning Juice Recipe** - 8-15 carrots (depending on size) & 1 Grapefruit (peeled). You're trying to make approximately 20oz - 32oz of juice. You don't have to chug it all, but try to drink it within an hour because the longer it sits, the more it "oxidizes" and changes the flavor and lowers nutritionally.

If buying juice instead, stay away from fruit heavy juices and no smoothies. This is all about nutrition, and I want you to get extra doses of veggies. Suja is a good brand of market available juices. Naked makes a decent all carrot juice. Odwalla brand is the last resort because they are ultra pasteurized which destroys a lot of the nutrition. Bolthouse brand carrot juice I can barely drink, their other juices are better tasting.

> **Lunch** - Pack a lunch if you can. If you can't do that, then change where and what you eat. The point of this is to change everything. It's only for the week so do your best. If you're up for the challenge, and you're healthy enough just juice lunch as well. Otherwise add juice to your packed lunch. I chose a green drink with lots of green leafy vegetables like kale and spinach and try to get some lemon and ginger into the mix.
>
> **Lunch Juice Recipe:** 1 Bunch of Kale, 2 hands full of Spinach, 1 apple, 1 lemon, 1 inch ginger

> **Dinner** - Change it up. Whatever you usually eat, do something different. NO EATING OUT. I want

you to cook your food regardless of your abilities. Watch a video if you have to. If you're juicing both breakfast and lunch, you're probably really hungry at this point. Don't overeat, take your time and only have 1 plate of food. No "Second" helping. You got all the nutrition you need for the day with the juice, so this is about calories, protein, and fat to satisfy you for sleeping.

EXERCISE

Whatever you chose to do from last week do that this week. Find one or two things to do that will take a minimum of 1 hour to complete at a moderate pace. Limit your intensity and focus on having fun. If you're jogging for 30 minutes, then plan to do some stretching or cool down walking after. The idea is to enjoy one hour of exercise.

GO TO BED EARLY THIS WEEK!

You're body will need the extra sleep, and it will help you not to overeat.

There is tremendous value in getting rest, and if you've worked hard this week and made a lot of changes it's really the best thing that you can do to keep up with the success of all the changes.

This week, we are developing new core belief tools that our sub-conscious will use for us moving forward. This week we are setting up the all important "Create" week. Do not skimp on getting sleep, adding extra nutrition, and changing everything you can. It's supposed to feel different and awkward. Be intentional about making these changes and decisions.

WEEK 3: CREATE
The Sweet Tooth &
Daily Short Exercise

The single worst enemy of having a healthy lifestyle are sweets. I love good cookies, I love bad cookies, heck I just really enjoy cookies. I know that eating them will not feel great the next day and it sets me backward. But, sometimes I "need" a cookie. I know that when I'm desperate for some junk food that it means I have an emotional need that isn't getting met. Just knowing that, allows me to either skip the junk and process the emotion; or go ahead and have the cookie and not spiral out of control into a 6-week junk food binge like it used to.

Having said that, once you get into the sweets your body will crave more of them, so it is an uphill battle. It takes 7 days to fully eliminate cravings for sweet foods. Once you get past that, you'll be amazed how you don't even want it.

It's time to fully accept a new way of living. You are forever going to be healthy and enjoy your life. This doesn't mean that you will never be allowed to have junk food or things that are obviously not good for you, it just means that you don't need them. For some a monthly chocolate fix is necessary, so don't sweat it and have a small very expensive piece of quality chocolate. Don't get caught stuffing yourself with things you don't want to avoid having that one thing that you do want. Just acknowledge that there is a reason behind it and either deal with that reason or skip the junk.

HERE ARE SOME GOOD TRICKS TO AVOIDING SUGAR IN OUR DAILY LIFE

No sweet drinks of any kind. - There is a slight caveat here, and that is if you are doing the juicing (you should be juicing vegetables mostly) they can be sweet, and that is the only exception.

If you have a morning coffee drink and you usually do so with sweetener then ditch all forms of sweetener. No sugar, sweet-n-low, stevia, or honey; just have your coffee with milk or whatever, and that's it.

Sweet tea is a tough one for many people, but it causes heart disease, so it's not worth it. Just have iced tea with no sweetener of any kind.

No diet sodas or fake sweeteners. If you're going to have something sweet make it the real stuff, it's way better for you than the fake stuff.

Salty for Sweet. Anytime you're thinking about getting a sweet treat or snack replace it for something salty. Salted nuts are good, and popcorn is good as well. Get the kind you pop yourself not microwaveable, (try to avoid junk potato chips and things like that), a piece of cheese can be good, anything salty will help break the sweet tooth.

Avoid sweet sauces. No sweet salad dressing, no sweet barbecue sauce, etc. Eventually this won't matter as much, but in the beginning, just avoid them to help yourself out.

ESCAPE CLAUSE: If you absolutely MUST

HAVE A SWEET then eat a piece of fruit. No dipping sauce or anything added. You can have a banana, apple, orange, grapes or whatever. Dried fruit is great as well, but some of those have added sugar so make sure you check the packaging. Dried cranberries and most dried mango slices are two culprits with added sugar.

This Week

28 Day No Sugar Challenge - That's right, it's challenge week. This week I want you to focus on killing the sweet tooth. I want you to continue this no sweets thing for 28 days. If it's the holidays, then you should wait until December 26th to start this.

Do your very best and DO NOT have any shame about messing up. You are learning right now, and it's important to be able to move on if you forget and have a little something.

THE NEXT 28 DAYS ARE LIKE A SCORE, NOT A SOBRIETY CHECK

Every day without sweets is worth 1 point. If you were offered sweets and you turned it down then take 2 points for that day.

Add up your score at the end of 28 days and post your Sweet Score in the Facebook group. Or anywhere you want and challenge someone else to match or beat your score.

56 points is a perfect score

28+ points is a great score

21-28 points is good

15-20 is not so good

Less than 15 is a do over, but it's a nice do over. :)

Don't worry about it; mistakes happen, this is supposed to be fun!

EXERCISE

28 Day Exercise Challenge - Start doing a daily exercise. Something simple that takes 15-30 minutes maximum. The idea here is to get into a healthy habit. Here are some that you can start, but feel free to find your own and go for it.

QUICK EXERCISES

60/60 - Every 60 minutes do an exercise for 60 seconds and string this together 5-8 times per day 5 days in a row.

Push-up's, Sit-up's/Crunches, Squats, Planks, Burpee's and Lunges are all great exercises that you can do anywhere even at work.

(See the charts on pg. 159-161)

Jogging - Head out your front door and go for a quick 20-30 min jog. It's easy and doesn't require anything more than a good pair of shoes. It's also something you can do during a lunch break, or if you are in a high-stress environment, it's a great way to end your work day before heading home. It doesn't have to be high intensity but doing it every day will help you a ton.

Stretching Break - Yoga is popular these days, but any general purpose stretching is great for you. It's quick easy and can be done anywhere without any equipment. Spend 15-30 minutes stretching and breathing. It's great for every exercise that you do to be limber, and it promotes blood flow to all parts of your body and clears cortisol. I like to end my day watching a little something on TV and stretching at the same time.

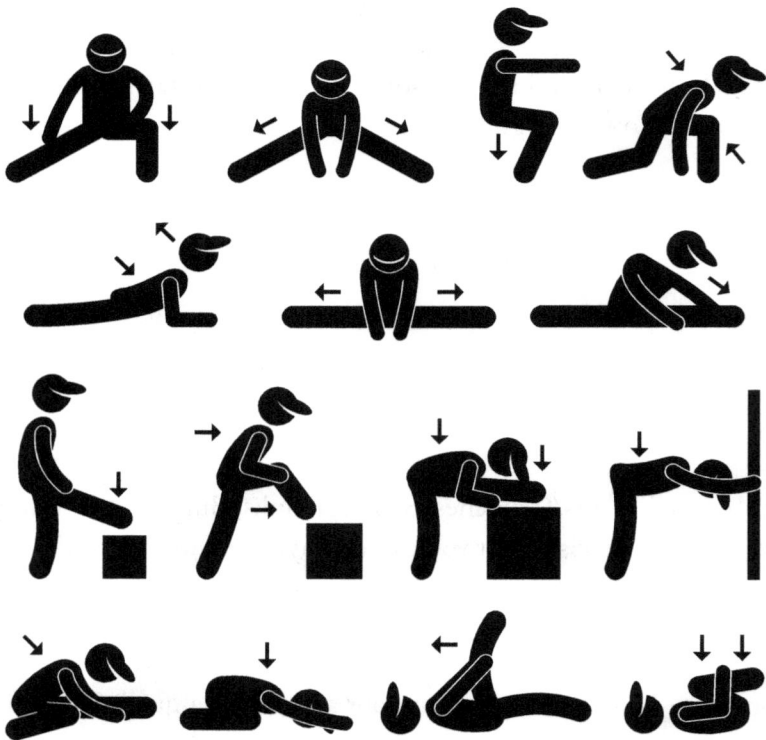

Jump Rope - Yes, and old fashioned jump rope is a great full body exercise, and you can do it in as little as 10 minutes per day. Also, it makes you feel kind of like a kid, so there's the added "fun" bonus. Jumping exercises, in general, are fantastic for your body.

Trampoline - Take a little trip on the trampoline, and you'll be amazed at the amount of fitness it takes to jump for 15-30 minutes. Some companies have built their entire business on trampoline fitness. You don't have to have a huge backyard bouncer; just a small personal trampoline is great. They range in price from $25 up to hundreds so just take a look at the weight specs and think about the amount of jumping you may do on it.

QUICK SIMPLE BODY WEIGHT EXERCISES

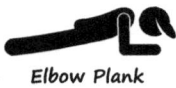
Elbow Plank

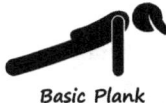
Basic Plank

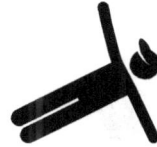
Elevated Side Plank

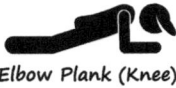
Elbow Plank (Knee)

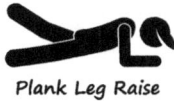
Plank Leg Raise

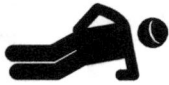
Bent Knee Side Plank

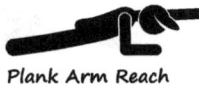
Plank Arm Reach

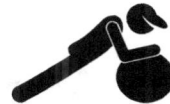
Ball Plank

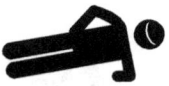
Side Plank

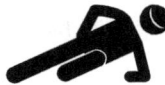
Side Plank
Knee Tuck (1)

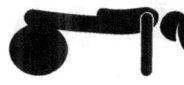
Ball Plank Reverse

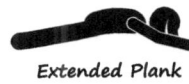
Extended Plank

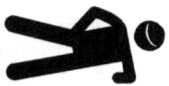
Side Plank Leg Lift

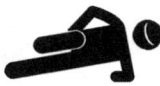
Side Plank
Knee Tuck (2)

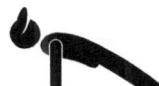
Reverse Plank

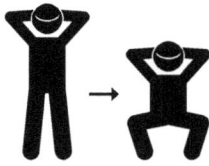

Bodyweight Squats

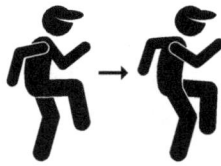

High Knees

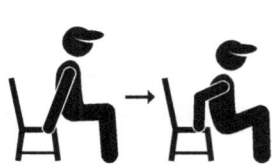

Chair Dips

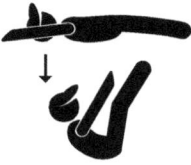

Toe Crunches

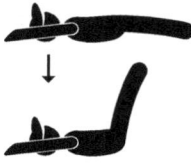

Leg Raises

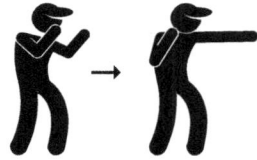

Punches

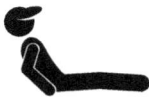

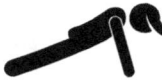

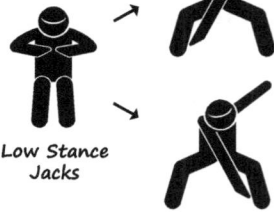

Knees Pull-Ins

Mountain Climbers

Low Stance Jacks

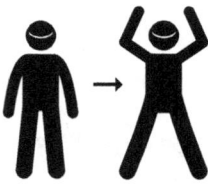

Jumping Jacks

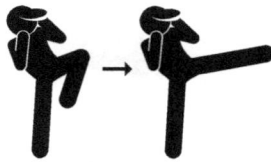

Side Kick

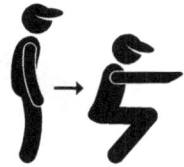

Squatting

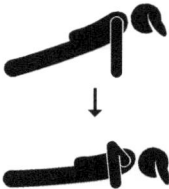

Push-up

Rotation

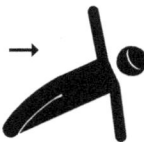

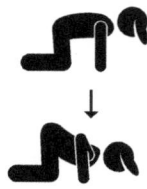

Knee Bent Push-up

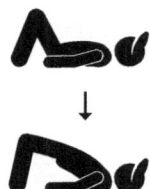

Pelvic Scoop

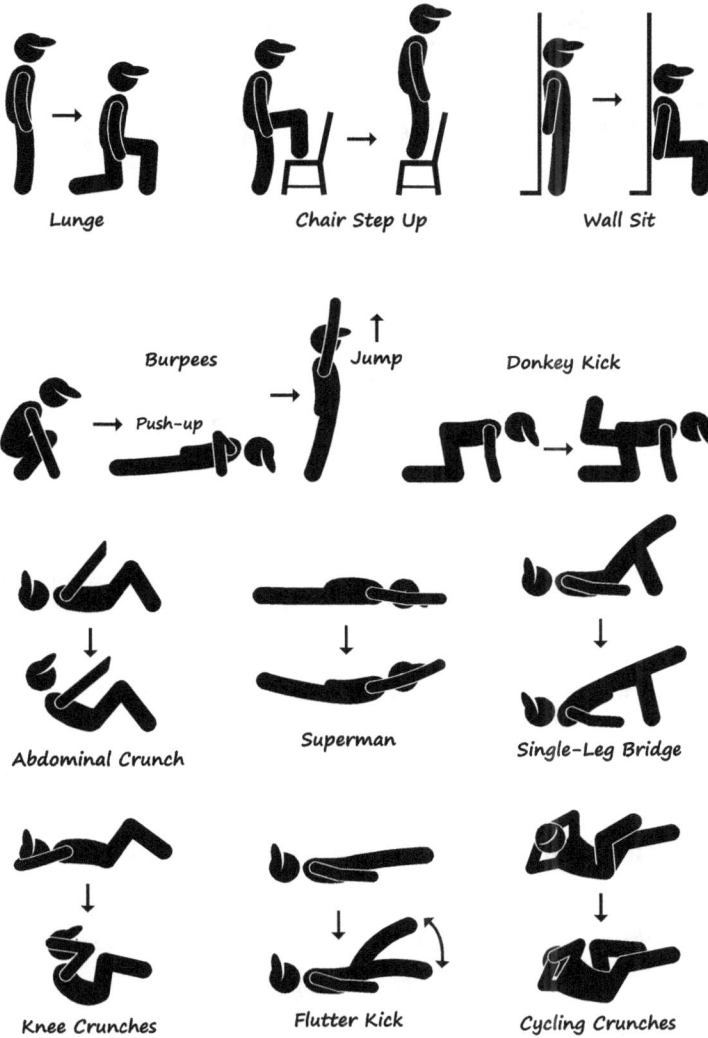

Lunge

Chair Step Up

Wall Sit

Burpees

Push-up

Jump

Donkey Kick

Abdominal Crunch

Superman

Single-Leg Bridge

Knee Crunches

Flutter Kick

Cycling Crunches

These are some basic exercises that you can do anywhere anytime. I like to do these for 60 seconds every hour while I'm at work. It refreshes the brain, makes me more productive, and helps get me fit at the same time. By the end of the day I have done 500 push-ups.

WEEK 4: SUCCESS
Plan for Someone Else

I enjoy helping other people find success. As a matter of fact, it's WAY easier to help someone else with their problem than it is to deal with my problem. This week is going to be simple. We are going to use the principle of helping someone else to help ourselves.

Think about a character, and give them a name. Then give them all your qualities. I want you to create some backstory for them (Try giving them your backstory). Then imagine that they come to you for advice on how to solve their weight problem. Diagnose them, and provide them with a diet and simple exercise plan that you think they can accomplish. Imagine you're asking them about their eating habits during the day, and their exercise, or lack thereof. Find out what's in their pantry and decide if those are good things or bad things to have.

- **Eliminate all junk food and quick eats like microwaveable stuff.**
- **Plan for healthy snacks, like fruit and a slice of cheese.**
- **Eliminate as many preservatives as possible.**
- **Plan cook from scratch meals for Breakfast, Lunch & Dinner.**
- **Eat breakfast!**

You've read the book on having fun with your weight loss journey, so nothing is strict. Everything is designed to aid in getting the best results.

I know this is somewhat basic, but it's very effective. Another way to do it is to plan as though you were helping your kids with a weight problem. Would you let them have that cookie? What would you pack for their lunch? What can they drink and what time should the go to bed? If they tell you they don't feel like doing the workout you have scheduled for them how would/should you respond?

Now, do that plan for yourself. AND STICK TO IT!

This Week

Create the person you're going to help and be detailed about their plan. You are potentially saving their life so be honest and meticulous. (This is the part where you get to chuckle)

1. **Do the plan you created for the "Made-Up Person"**
2. **Share your results with someone you trust, or everyone via social media.**

This is supposed to be a fun experiment to give you insight into the things you may not be doing well and to reveal how much you know. If you come across something that you just can't get rid of, ask yourself why? Is it something that you need to get over or is it something that you really enjoy and are willing to leave in your life.

Smile through the process!

Chapter 11
THE WRAP UP

Are you living your life or is your life living you?

One of the biggest struggles when trying to slay the weight demon is confusion around biology and identity. Your biology is not your current physique. Regardless of whether you are an ideal weight or 100 pounds overweight, your biology is the same. You are the same person with the same DNA. Forcing an identity out of being overweight is one of the main reasons you're stuck.

BIOLOGY & IDENTITY

Identity has two main parts, Core and External. Your core identity cannot be changed or disputed, but your external identity is created and is completely a choice. Saying, "I am fat;" is the same as saying that it's impossible for you ever to be thin or even a healthy weight.

When your physique creates the identity of being "a fat person," it takes away the option ever to be "normal." Neither your physique or your external identity have anything to do with your biology or your core identity. Learning to embrace your core identity and the biology is the doorway to freedom.

Some parts of biology do connect to core identity. I am tall. I am blue eyed. I am a mesomorph. Because of this truth, it becomes easy to form core identity around what we see in the mirror.

The Questions:

- "What lies are you believing about yourself?"
- Is your current body shape stealing your hope?
- Do you believe that you were born the way you look now?
- Is it harder for you than other people?

Don't believe any statement that keeps you stuck. There is always hope. Search on YouTube for people in your same condition that got out of it. Everyone has the power to create the life they want. Even if you're currently starting at a point further away than someone else, where you end is completely up to you. Everything you need to be the person you've always wanted is available to those who accept it.

OVEREATING

One of the leading causes of overeating is a lack of CONNECTION. In fact, one of the main reasons for all compulsions or addictions is a lack of connection. There are three kinds of connection that are important.

Personal - Spouse, Children, Immediate Family and close friends.

Social - Social interaction is one of pillars of personal needs.

Internal - If you're not connected to your own heart then everything you do will be challenging, including losing weight and keeping it off.

I've heard people say, "I wish I didn't have to eat alone" and I get that it's not always possible to be with people when you're eating. Even saying this can cause some pain for a portion of you but ultimately unless we learn how to connect in these three areas it will be more challenging than it has to. If relationship is a sore spot for you, join a lunch networking group or just frequent a local coffee shop during lunch time. You won't always be able to eat with others, but it's a great practice to find ways to connect. Invite people over for dinner and keep it simple. Go to breakfast with friends or do whatever you can.

Ultimately it's not about eating, it's about connecting. Join a workout group, or a walking club or any special interest group and be intentional about connecting with others. Most people are not great at connecting, so it takes work to do that but it's worth it. Don't be needy about it, just be intentional about loving people well and it will reciprocate.

NUTRITION IS A JOURNEY

Food is supposed to be a fun journey. I love to eat, and I really enjoy discovering new foods and reminiscing with old classics. Learning how to eat healthy is a journey and the best way to deal with it is a little at a time. Pick one thing like replacing your unhealthy snacking with a healthy version. You're supposed to have fun with your "diet." I suggest staying away from extreme nutrition programs but ultimately you're going to have to decide for yourself what's going to work.

The Fun Diet Nutrition Program - Eat a healthy balanced high vegetable & high nutrition diet; that's it.

Your body needs food, all of it, including carbs and fats. We actually don't need as much protein as most people eat. We don't need to overload on food. Being intentional about eating smaller quality meals that are high in nutrition is the hallmark of a healthy lifestyle.

1. Eat breakfast no matter what, even if it's small or simple but always eat breakfast.

2. Eliminate junk food from your normal daily routine but be ok with having something special every once in awhile. No pressure, just know that every bite of junk food is sending you in the wrong direction.

3. Don't eat late. Be done after dinner, or if you know you're going to be awake more than 4hrs after your "last meal" then eat a bit less at dinner and keep the late snack "tiny" because you only need to cut the craving.

Have fun with diving into all the cool things about food. Get a dehydrator, a juicer, sprouting jars, and a really good blender. Learn how to use them and make some amazing foods! It's so fun to tell people that we buy grains and sprout them, then dehydrate them, then grind them into flour. It doesn't take as much work as it sounds, and it really is fun!

The Fun Exercise Program - Play! Find things that are a blast, and do them. Sports, group exercises, even running around with your kids. Life is too short not to enjoy your exercise. Get out and hike! Whatever you find in your heart to do, do it! Try everything until you find something that you really enjoy. I discovered that I love to swim, and that it's really fun to road bike. You never know until you try.

> **Daily:** find short 15-30 min exercises that you can do daily to grow your overall health.

> **Weekly:** find one thing at minimum that takes 1hour or more of exercising.
>
> Annually: A couple of times a year, find something really hard to do and go for it! A marathon, a mud race, or a backpacking trip. It doesn't matter what you do but set goals throughout the year that will help you stay on track with exercising regularly.

> Regular exercise is a must! Not just for your physical wellbeing but also for your mental and emotional health. It's important that we don't get stuck indoors. Even if it's cold or raining or whatever, get outside and enjoy it. Embrace the beauties of where you live.

THE BEST VERSION OF YOU

Imagine what the best version of you would be like. Don't focus on the physical aspect. Think about the kinds of activities you participate in and the kinds of fun you have. Think about what you do for a living, and where you live. Now take steps towards doing those things. The world needs your special qualities in it. We need to be encouraged by your strength and passions. The Fun Diet is focused on building people up to be full of passion and connected to their own hearts. We're using the struggle with weight to get you to that place, but in the end it's the only way to truly be free from the shame and challenge of dieting and being overweight.

DON'T BE SO HARD ON YOURSELF

Typically, we are our worst critics. Take it easy, if you're having a rough season it's acceptable to notice that you're not making good choices. The sooner you can see it, and recognize what you need to do differently, the sooner you can get back on track. Being hard yourself will only perpetuate the problem. You're human and you have needs beyond just physical so often you will do harmful things to your body because you have emotional needs that you're trying to fix with food. Food won't solve your problem, and it's a bandaid but give yourself a break when you blow it and get back on track quickly.

FUN WITH FRIENDS

Life is better when shared. Bring someone along with you on this journey. Not everyone will be as excited as you are, but it's really fun to have a friend to share the challenge with. The point of life is to have fun in connection with others so make this an intentional part of losing weight and enjoying the process.

THE END

Life is a gift, and it's worth living well. It may not be all your fault for where you are today but where you are tomorrow is completely up to you. You are the master of your fate. It's time to take responsibility for the things in your life that you can change and start moving forward toward goals that make you happy.

"Life is either a daring adventure or nothing at all"
- Helen Keller

BONUS CHALLENGES

Without challenges, you will forget how
awesome you are.

I t takes 21-28 days to create a habit. Challenging yourself to do new things for 28 days is a great way to start healthy habits. Try some of these or come up with your own challenges and have fun!

LEMON WATER CHALLENGE - Every day for 28 days

start your day with a full glass of lemon water. Squeeze ½ a lemon or whatever you can stand into a 12oz glass of water then drink it before you start your day. Lemons have an amazing property where the type of "acid" in them when processed through the body will carry the bad acids that are hanging around with them on the way out. So even though a lemon is acidic the acid in them will help make you ph neutral or alkaline. #LemonWaterChallenge

MARATHON CHALLENGE - 28 days in a row run 1 mile

or more. Rain or shine, sick or healthy get outside and run 1 mile every day for 28 days straight. Can you do it? #MarathonChallenge

DO NEW CHALLENGE - Do something new for 28 days

in a row. It can be cooking a new food you've never tried before or doing some new exercise that you've never tried before. Get creative but keep it in the realm of health and fitness. #DoNewChallenge

SUGAR CHALLENGE - How long can you go without sugar? Challenge yourself to a minimum of 28 days sugar free. Having fake sugar in doesn't count. We're talking about any added sugar. A piece of fruit is ok, but anything with added sugar in it isn't allowed. Can you go 365 days in a row? #SugarChallenge

JUICING CHALLENGE - Get a juicer and juice 28 days in a row. Use it as a meal replacement or in addition to what you're eating. The goal is to supercharge your nutrition for 28 days. You will be amazed at how good you feel. Focus on juicing vegetables but you can add fruits to help build great flavors. #JuicingChallenge

HAPPINESS CHALLENGE - I created a 28 day challenge with unique things to do everyday to boost your happiness quotient. Go to ryan8.com/happy28 and start the program for free. It's a great way to boost your happy body chemicals which adds to everything you do including losing weight. #HappinessChallenge

BREATHING CHALLENGE - Deep breathing is super beneficial for your health. Can you spend 28 days in a row just breathing without thinking of what else you should be doing? Day 1 you will breath deeply with your eyes closed for 1 minute. Day 2 you will breath for 2 minutes, and day 3 three minutes. Every day you will be adding 1 minute to your time. See if you can make it to 28 minutes in a row of quiet breathing. I choose to sit in meditation with God, not praying just being. The breathing without thinking about the things that you need to do is the goal, so if you have trouble in silence just focus on your breathing. Think about the breath coming in and the breath going out. Set a timer if you have to so you don't need to think about the time. #BreathingChallenge

NEGATIVITY CHALLENGE - Fast from all negativity for 28 days. That may mean staying away from your favorite TV show that isn't uplifting or avoiding conversations with certain people. As much as possible avoid all negativity for 28 days in a row. Including using negative statements like: I can't, I won't, I'm not able to, etc... Focus on using positive statements instead. #NegativityChallenge

It can help to make a list of your bad habits.

ELIMINATE BAD HABIT

1

2

3

4

5

6

7

8

9

10

Then take the list of bad habits and find replacements for them.

REPLACE WITH GOOD HABIT

1

2

3

4

5

6

7

8

9

10

ABOUT THE AUTHOR

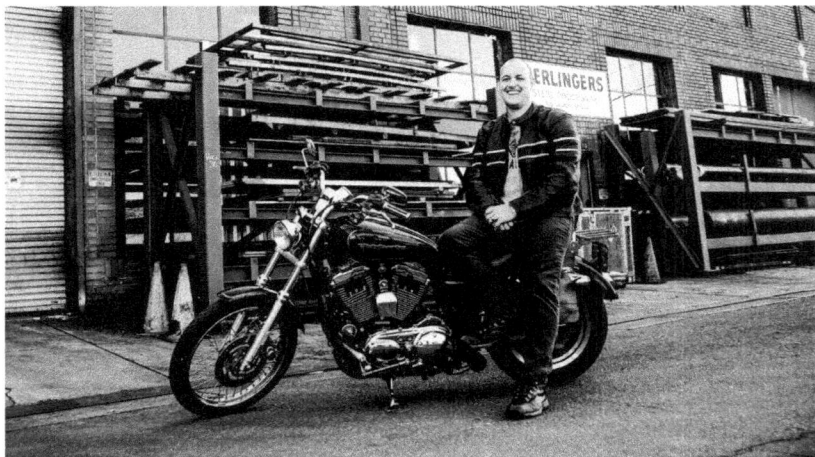

RYAN ANDREWS is a business owner, speaker, consultant and entrepreneur. He was the co-host of a #1 comedy podcast and a #1 psychology podcast. He is a worship pastor of over 17 years and has been all over the world helping people find their passion. His pursuit is to represent a life on fire.

Ryan is one of those people that you meet and immediately want to engage. He has learned through a lifetime of overcoming challenges how to enjoy life to the fullest and he discovered that his passion is helping others to find what makes them come alive. He has completed the Ironman 70.3 triathlon in Lake Tahoe, and is an endurance athlete competing in olympic distance and cross country triathlons. He is currently training to climb Mt. Kilimanjaro.

Ryan grew up in Hawaii, and lives in Redding, CA with his beautiful wife Nissa, and their 4 children.

www.ryan8.com

FREEBIES

Download Worksheets & Notes
www.ryan8.com/fundietws

Ryan's 60/60 Workout Plan
www.ryan8.com/fundietwp

28 Days of Happy Challenge
ryan8.com/happy28

Facebook
www.facebook.com/fundietbook

Private Support Group
www.facebook.com/groups/fundiet

Website
www.Ryan8.com/fundiet

I would love to hear from all of you.

Visit the website www.ryan8.com and send me a message.

www.ingramcontent.com/pod-product-compliance
Lightning Source LLC
Chambersburg PA
CBHW071126280326
41935CB00010B/1130